Emmanuel Cauchy is one of the world's top mountain-rescue doctors. He worked as medical advisor on such films as *Himalaya*, and *James Bond – Tomorrow Never Dies*. His principal work is in the French Alps, where for the last twenty years he has served with the PGHM, the helicopter mountain rescue covering the Chamonix and Mont Blanc region. He also coordinates IFREMMONT, the Institute for Training and Research in Mountain Medicine, of which he is a founder member.

HANGING BY A THREAD

HANGING BY A THREAD

THE MISSIONS OF A HELICOPTER RESCUE DOCTOR

EMMANUEL CAUCHY

Translated by Jo Cleere

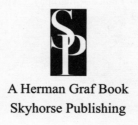

A Herman Graf Book
Skyhorse Publishing

Skyhorse Publishing books may be purchased in bulk at special discounts for sales promotion, corporate gifts, fund-raising, or educational purposes. Special editions can also be created to specifications. For details, contact the Special Sales Department, Skyhorse Publishing, 555 Eighth Avenue, Suite 903, New York, NY 10018 or info@skyhorsepublishing.com.

www.skyhorsepublishing.com

10 9 8 7 6 5 4 3 2 1

Library of Congress Cataloging-in-Publication Data

Cauchy, Emmanuel, 1960-
  [Petit manuel de médecine de montagne. English]
  Hanging by a thread : the missions of a helicopter rescue doctor / Emmanuel Cauchy ; translated by Jo Cleere.
      p. cm.
  ISBN 978-1-60239-659-3
  1. Cauchy, Emmanuel, 1960- 2. Mountaineering injuries--Blanc, Mont (France and Italy) 3. Mountaineering accidents--Blanc, Mont (France and Italy) 4. Rescue work--Blanc, Mont (France and Italy) 5. Emergency physicians--France--Biography. I. Title.
  RC88.9.M6C38 2009
  617.1'027092--dc22
  [B]
  2008054412

Printed in England

To Jacotte, my mother, and my father Jean-Pépé,
'the master mariner', and owner of the boat I sank.

To Cécile, Pierrot, Alix and Khando.

To the Big Chief.

And to Don Quixote!

CONTENTS

• • • • • • • • •

Author's note   xi

Prologue   xiii

1 MEMORIES

A First Blow   3

Welcome to the Drop Zone   13

Danger-man   20

2 WINTER

Blue Cathedral   31

The Slender Thread   44

A Different Kind of Rescue   63

Big Chief   67

Blades in the Snow   84

Jamie   97

Frostbite at the North Pole   104

Blood on The Mountain   111

3 SUMMER

Gervasutti Pillar: Friday   129

The Dead Guy's Not Dead   136

White Death   149

Gervasutti Pillar: The Storm   165

Marvels of Modern Technology   173

Gervasutti Pillar: End in Sight   184

Pawns of Fate   189

Feeling the Heat   210

A Walk in the Park   232

Alive   248

In Doctors' Hands   257

Better than Vegas   266

Epilogue   278

AUTHOR'S NOTE

• • • • • • • • •

This is a book based on real events, though some names have been changed. It is an autobiography which I am dedicating to my colleagues, most of whom will no doubt recognize themselves in these pages. I hope they will see my portrayal of them in these stories as a reflection of the profound sense of friendship I feel, and will remember with me those moments of struggle that united us in the face of adversity.

My respect for those who survived, and those who did not, and who provided me with the material for this collection of rescue accounts is immeasurable. I found motivation in all of their stories to persevere and bring recognition to our profession. This book is a tribute to those who devoted their lives to rescues, and who were taken from us while doing their job – to my friends who have died almost in front of my eyes in the mountains.

EC

PROLOGUE

● ● ● ● ● ● ● ● ●

When I was little I wanted to be a vet. I loved animals and, apart from two or three cowardly mutts attacking my ankles from behind, they liked me too. I used to gather up sick birds, even the terminal cases, and make them swallow aspirin with absolutely no notion of such things as toxic doses. Few survived.

Once, my father and I built a cage in the corner of the dining room to keep quails. It's amazing how bad they smell. If only they could whistle or tweet, and they're not even very graceful in flight. There were feathers and bits of grit everywhere except in the cage and I fear my mother had a hand in their suspected poisoning.

After struggling my way though the grades that would, in theory, open the doors of the baccalauréat to me, and having learnt of the unavoidable and stringent selection process used by the veterinary schools, I decided to set my sights on a more modest goal: treating patients of the human variety. I was always more practical than intellectual, so I thought I'd give surgery a go as that was my uncle's field and he didn't seem to mind groping around inside his patients for a living.

I scraped through my bac and got into medical school on my second attempt, to the great surprise of my parents who expected me to end up in a football team.

While my brain struggled with ill-digested chunks of photo-copies and handouts, I devoted a great deal of time and energy to sailing. I had been sailing since I was a boy and was a mariner at heart, spending my time navigating the waters of the Channel in search of adventure. I was probably too cocky the time I really got out of my depth.

That day my friend Michel and his brother joined me to sail in the waters off Cabourg, and I narrowly missed sending us all to the bottom. We braved the spray to end up a few nautical miles off the coast. We energetically steered the little 470, the boat I'd borrowed from my father, as it heaved up and down in the swell that showed no signs of abating. Our dinghy was hardly the last word in boat design. More and more white horses were forming and slamming into its hull. Michel's brother wasn't much of a sailor but he was pretty tough and, more importantly, he had us in stitches. He was such a good laugh that for his initiation we decided to introduce him to tra-pezing, counteracting the boat's heel by sitting in a harness on a wire attached to the mast. He didn't have his sea legs and every time a wave hit he was sent flying, getting a face full of water for his troubles.

I was a little distracted by all the monkeying around and after we had been at sea for about an hour, it dawned on me that the boat was filling up with water faster than it was drain-ing away and the waterline was unusually low. Our efforts at bailing it out weren't working. All of a sudden the coast looked very far away indeed and the atmosphere onboard changed completely.

We brought the boat about to try to head for land but it slowly started to sink and we realized the seriousness of our predicament. I silently ran through the technical reasons why modern materials made this kind of boat virtually unsinkable and decided that the only way to drain the water from it was to capsize her. It was also the only way of signalling to the rescue teams, supposedly keeping a lookout, that there was something wrong.

Fat chance! Half an hour later we still hadn't seen anyone. The bozos in charge of surveillance were obviously catching up on all the week's papers, paragraph by paragraph.

My two companions were excellent swimmers and set off for the shore doing the front crawl. Convinced that a captain should never leave his ship, I grabbed hold of a sheet and waited for the rescue I still thought was coming. Twenty minutes later I was in water up to my neck. Only the bottom of the dinghy was still poking above the surface, like an iceberg, and I was treading water trying not to freeze to death.

I managed to get on to the boat's upturned belly to see if I could spot anything over the mountainous waves. After a great deal of squirming I was able to stand up rather precariously, and I finally spotted them. There were my mates, scarcely 200 metres from the boat. Everything – the life jackets, the current and the waves – was hampering their progress.

I slid back into the water and it suddenly hit me: the boat was probably going to sink and if it did, it would take me down with it. I had to get out of there. It felt like I swam for hours. I had got into a rhythm but I knew I wasn't getting anywhere and I tried not to think about it. Yet the reality of the situation was blindingly obvious: I would finish up sinking to the bottom, utterly exhausted. I sensed the hundreds of metres of black water and nothingness beneath my feet and I was terrified. The vertigo was as bad as if I was suspended over a huge chasm.

My agonizing was interrupted by the sounds of a motor and shouting. A Zodiac, which happened to be passing through, had picked up my friends and they had come looking for me. I will never know what kind of miracle led them to me.

The boat was gone, my dad was furious and I started a new chapter in my life. I decided to devote my time to the mountains

1

MEMORIES

· · · · · · · · ·

A FIRST BLOW

• • • • • • • • •

We tend to think that climbers tempting fate on terrifying cliffs have something of a do-or-die attitude. They are often young and determined, and accept the risks involved. Wunderkind climbers who have been training hard from an early age seem to be scampering up the most difficult routes around these days, routes which used to take experienced guides several days to climb. There are still the same dangers involved but, as we tend to talk of those who survive rather than those who don't make it, this is not always obvious. It often only dawns on us when we have children of our own, who are starting to do the same bloody stupid things themselves.

I should know what I'm talking about, as I used to be just like them. Obviously I didn't die but I had several close calls. Some were so close that I'm inclined to think that there's a third way, between doing and dying, that's called the reality check. In the mountains this is something that takes you, your ego and any illusions you might have of your own abilities down a peg or two. A good metaphorical slap in the face will keep you alive.

I remember my first close call as if it were yesterday. My friend Michel and I had diligently put together a pretty stringent training regime. We were getting more and more into the mountains, devoting ourselves to them; training on bits of cliffs, having aerial jousting matches in hang-gliders, and ski touring in the Chablais, no matter the weather. Whenever our days off coincided we would head for the mountains.

This particular winter we had climbed the north face of the Courtes in the Mont Blanc range with disconcerting ease and in record time. The descent was particularly good fun, as we had glissaded down 800 metres of snow clutching our ice axes, hoping they would stop us if need be. Instead of the two hours it would have taken us if we had stayed roped together, we reached our skis in just fifteen minutes, as pleased as Punch. We felt ready for anything.

Convinced we were sufficiently experienced to have a go at something more serious, Michel suggested we try the north face of the Matterhorn before having a crack at the Eiger! Michel's main failing was that he was too sure of himself, whereas I lacked self-confidence. Between the two of us there lay a happy medium.

So off we set to conquer the legendary north face of the Matterhorn.

The morning of our memorable climb saw two other pairs set on doing the same route as us, standing at the foot of the face. The forecast couldn't have been better: high pressure had brought blue skies and cold dry weather. The ice conditions, however, weren't so great, as we soon discovered. The first section of the climb, a steep snowfield, was covered in glassy black ice and the first team, just in front of us, had already turned back. The other team, in an attempt to overtake the first group, had started further along. After only fifty metres the leader gave up, his calf muscles screaming, abandoning an ice screw so his partner could lower him down.

We were now the only team on the face. We assumed this to be down to our superior climbing skills but it soon proved to be a Pyrrhic victory. The die had been cast right from the moment we first set foot on the route proper: we had to carry on. There were no tracks, no evidence of belay stances and it didn't seem at all obvious which way to go on this supposedly really well-known route.

The first 300 metres were rotten and dangerous, nothing like the north face of the Courtes. The ice was thin and we never knew which line to follow, forced to constantly weave our way between loose rocks and sections of ice. As there weren't many decent protection placements and in an effort to save time, we decided to move together. There were hardly any solid spikes of rock to hang slings on and we never had more than three pieces of protection between us. Even then, they wouldn't have held a fall and were there more for psychological support than any actual physical protection. After just two hours of climbing we were knackered. Our packs weighed a ton and the route seemed to go on forever. We had taken loads of risks and had climbed a good third of the face. We had been swapping leads. Some of the tricky sections had me scared stiff, as I knew we simply wouldn't survive a fall. Michel, who climbed at the same level as me, was encountering the same problems and was feeling the pressure as much as I was. Yet I had complete faith in him, as he kept his cool in tricky situations.

At around 10 a.m. we allowed ourselves a break to assess our predicament. It was the first decent stance we had found all day. We hadn't spoken much since setting off and now we really needed to talk!

'We're gonna get ourselves bloody killed, Michel! The rock's totally rotten.'

'Yeah. I think we've gone too far left …'

'You sure?'

'Well, not completely, it's difficult to know where we are now.'

'I'm not feeling too good. We're not acclimatized for this altitude.'

'No, I suppose not.'

We scrutinized the outline of the northeast ridge 150 metres above our heads. The escape route we had picked out earlier on was up there somewhere. It would be suicidal to try and abseil down a face like this with no proper stances.

'Are you thinking what I'm thinking, Michel?'

'Yeah, I think that's the safest option. I'm happy to leave the route, it's not in condition. Shame though, the weather's pretty stable,' he added with a hint of regret.

'We should be able to get to the Solvay hut without too much difficulty. We'll have to take the little gully on the left, then follow the normal route down.'

We took a final look at our new line and resigned ourselves to our chosen course of action. The face steepened before joining the ridge but we could make out a gully with what looked like half-decent ice.

Michel said, 'Want to go first or am I belaying you?' which was our stock joke question for when things looked a bit dicey.

'It's my turn, I'll go.'

It was almost the biggest mistake of my life. Off I set with renewed impetus, comforted by the thought that we would soon be out of this mess. Ten metres higher up I clipped my rope into the first piton of the route, a rusty peg that stuck out of the rock by five centimetres. Twenty metres above this I managed, with difficulty, to place a small wire in a crack in the rock for protection but I didn't like the look of it. The gully steepened and, viewed up close, the ice covering it looked pretty dubious. There was no point exhausting myself trying to place ice screws in the rotten stuff here, and I headed for the sheet of more solid-looking ice above. The climbing was getting more and more committing but I reckoned I could get a really good ice screw placement up there.

As I got to the bottom of the sheet of ice I felt the first pangs of anxiety rising up inside me, which wasn't a good sign. The ice wasn't stuck to the rock at all. I had to climb up the rock pillar to the left, before rejoining the upper section of ice.

I was climbing at my limit and was becoming seriously exhausted. By the time I got to ten metres above the wire I had placed, I was really starting to freak out. Michel watched me like a hawk. He had known me for so long that I didn't have to say a word, he understood exactly what was happening.

There was one last delicate move right to get on to the sheet of ice. Once there, I found a stable position for my crampons and planted my axes in the ice above my head. I unclipped an ice screw from my harness and for a few seconds, as I watched it bite into the ice, I felt waves of relief wash through me. That is until the screw – I had deliberately chosen a long one – was halfway in the ice. At that point I heard a sinister cracking noise and felt the entire plate of ice I was on gently detach itself from the rock. I panicked and undid the ice screw by a single turn. Still panicking, I rushed to try and put my hand through the leash on my axe so I could escape as quickly as possible. It's always at moments like these, just when you don't want anything to go wrong, that cock-ups happen. My glove caught on the loop, stopping my hand going into it. Cursing the damned thing, I did what I was most trying to avoid: I let the axe slip through my hands. I heard the metallic sound of it tumbling over and over again, all the way down to the bottom of the face. Clutching my one remaining ice axe and powerless to react, I waited for the entire sheet of ice to peel away from the rock and hurl me into the abyss.

But it held. I had been given a second chance. My only way out now was to gingerly crawl on to the other side of the ice and get to a tiny nubbin of rock where I could set up a make-shift belay. I summoned up all my powers of concentration and managed by some kind of miracle to plant the edge of my arse on to a paltry lump of rock frozen into the ice. I had made it. I was physically exhausted and emotionally I was a nervous wreck. I felt like a castaway stranded on some monstrous iceberg.

'Fuuuuuuuuck, Michel!' I screamed at the top of my voice in an attempt to let off some nervous energy.

'Yeah,' came the reply from thirty-five metres below.

'I nearly bloody died! That's it. I'm done. I'm scared shit-less up here!'

I could see the two climbers from the second team, which had turned around, right at the bottom of the face. They were about 100 metres apart, taking it easy and having a picnic in the sun. I cursed myself for not having decided to turn round when we could, like they had done. All because we thought we were better than them!

And now what was I supposed to do? It was impossible to get any kind of protection into the rock, I couldn't even use my friends, as their springloaded cams would not hold in the totally rotten and crumbly surface. And we didn't have a radio.

The silence was broken by Michel shouting up to me.

'Manu, what do we do now?'

'I have no idea but I'm not going anywhere.'

'Can you set up a belay?'

'There's nothing. There's nothing but shitty rock on this fucking mountain.'

Never short of ideas, Michel realized he had a survival bag in his pack. He waved it around in the direction of the two climbers below us. Old-fashioned methods still have their uses. The other climbers must have heard the ice axe falling and were probably asking themselves if everything was ok. Ten minutes later we saw them set off in the direction of the Hörnli hut. We hoped they had understood.

The three-hour wait seemed interminable. We were in the shade and we were staying in the shade. Michel's ledge was a bit more comfortable than my one and he had put some extra clothes on. I, on other hand, couldn't move at all. I was terrified of losing my balance and didn't even dare take off my pack as it might have unbalanced me. In any case, there was nowhere to put it. I was frozen and shaking uncontrollably. The heat from my arse, on the other hand, was melting the ice that was holding the rock I was perched on in place and I could feel it slowly loosening.

Every quarter of an hour or so the sound of a motor would get up my hopes of a rescue. But they were planes doing tourist trips, the passengers idiotically waving at me. I could have killed them …

I felt myself slipping into a desperate torpor when all of a sudden a Lama helicopter appeared out of nowhere and whirled around us. When it came up close to us we realized it was a rescue helicopter. The pilot was making signs to me that seemed to mean: 'Are you the ones up shit creek?' I was shivering so much that I wasn't sure how much longer I could stay perched on my little rock. But the sight of the helicopter gave me a huge boost. Michel had his hands free and responded with the conventional signals letting them know we needed help. But the chopper flew off and we didn't see it again for another hour. Had they understood?

More sounds of engines and this time there were two helicopters: a Lama and an Ecureuil. We watched them whirling round in front of us as if they couldn't decide what to do. Then nothing. We were back to square one. This was wearing me down and I was just about ready to give up.

Another hour went by and the Lama was back. It hovered over my head and the downdraft from the rotor blades almost blew me off my tiny platform of rock. Just when I was expecting a cable to be lowered down to me, I saw a rescuer dangling above my head. I had no idea what he was planning to do or where the hell he thought he was going. I was terrified he was going to swing into me and knock me off my perch. I had only the haziest notion of how I thought they were going to rescue me. I thought they would drop a cable down to me, I would untie the rope attaching me to Michel and they would winch me into the chopper. But clearly they had decided to make it much more complicated.

The guy was being lowered down towards me and there was nothing I could do about it. He had an ice axe in his right hand

and two friends attached to his harness, and that was it! Either he was supremely confident and taking the piss, or he was about to be very scared indeed.

He set down next to me with his front points in a patch of rotten ice and placed his ice axe as best he could. He unclipped the cable from his harness and, instead of passing it to me so that I could be winched to safety, gave the ok sign to the helicopter. It flew off. What the hell was going on?

He talked to me in German, a language I have failed to master.

'*Kein piton? Kein piton?*' he shouted, trying to find somewhere to place the friends from his harness.

'*Nein, kein piton!*' was all I could reply.

At that moment I saw his right foot slip and the other one freeze where it was. I was sure he was only going to last another five seconds before falling off completely. I watched the colour drain from his face. A little hesitantly, given my own predicament, I held out my hand to help him. It was very possible he would take us both down. By some kind of miracle he managed to get his balance and I held on to him while he reached for his radio with his free hand and called the helicopter back.

Once again there was the wind tunnel of the chopper's rotor blades and the cable with its safety hook was lowered down to us. In a remarkably generous act of fair play, my rescuer handed the safety hook to me first. I clipped it into my harness, untied the rope and was winched away.

The feeling of happiness I had as I felt myself lifted up into the air at that moment will remain with me for the rest of my life. As I moved away from the face I realized just how frighteningly vertical it was and how serious the enterprise upon which we had embarked had actually turned out to be.

In less than two minutes I was standing in the sun in front of the hut. Michel landed next to me a quarter of an hour later. We looked at each other. We were safe and there was nothing more to be said.

It had been close.

I was so cold I couldn't speak a word without stammering. It took me an hour of warming up before I could even laugh. I was really disappointed but very, very happy. I would bless helicopters for the rest of my life.

WELCOME TO THE DROP ZONE

• • • • • • • • •

The boat at the bottom of the Channel and a degree in medicine in my pocket, there seemed to be only one course of action left open to me: become a specialist mountain doctor, save shepherdesses in distress and climb Everest! I had images of setting off in the middle of a stormy night up snowy Alpine slopes with climbing skins on my skis, rushing to the aid of some poor woman who had given birth unexpectedly.

After realizing that the majority of premature births take place in the ambulance on the way to the hospital, I got a place to do my military service at the École militaire de haute montagne (EMHM) in Chamonix as a trainee doctor. My work consisted in monitoring the health of the young recruits who, for better or for worse, had been drafted into the ranks to traipse across expanses of snow and ice, preferably two by two, with the sole purpose of being on duty and acting as punching-bags for small-minded officers.

That said, I have no regrets about my year of zealous military service. I learnt to pull the famous floppy *chasseur alpin* beret on my head and to get up to the sound of the early morning bugle call and a 'proud salute of light', as a young officer once told us. In short, I learnt to do nothing, but early in the morning!

During my military service I also got the opportunity to go on call for the first time with the Peloton de gendarmerie de haute montagne (PGHM), the mountain rescue team. The peloton is unique to Chamonix and is the leading authority in mountain rescues. It was made up of gendarmes who were also rescuers, and some could be pretty pig-headed and were more gendarme than rescuer. Thankfully, there were others who had chosen the job to be able to work in the mountains. They were more rescuers than gendarmes. Despite my initial reservations, I made some good friends in both camps. Whatever people said about them, their rigorous and severe nature went hand in hand with the work itself. Some were the kings of ropework and others were the masters of winching people off cliff faces. On the other hand, the helicopter was one of their principal modes of transport and I was staggered by the tiny number of rescues done on foot.

However, medically speaking things were pretty wide of the mark. This was still the heroic era of heli-stretchering, which consisted in bundling the victim up in a stretcher as quickly as possible and relying on the cold, wind and din of the helicopter to stifle their cries, before they were dumped at the nearest hospital. The medical support was equal to the means the medics were able to provide: that is to say, they didn't fly very high. It might sometimes be an ophthalmologist or perhaps a psychiatrist, for whom the mountains were the ideal place for existential self-interrogations, taking part in the rescue. That must have been a great comfort to the trauma victim! The docs were there for decoration, token medics wheeled out for ceremonial occasions.

In short, when I arrived in Chamonix, I was neither recognized for my skills as a mountaineer nor for my skills as an emergency doctor. This was mainly because emergency medicine was not taught as a subject back then and experience, 'the lamp one carries attached to one's back which only ever lights up the path already trod', was conspicuous by its absence from my CV. I had just finished studying and I was a novice. I don't know the exact circumstances that prompted the inclusion of a doctor in the rescue team, but I imagine a recent and rather delicate incident had forced the issue of the lack of medical care on to the agenda.

Unable to join the Chamonix hospital emergency department, I managed to get contract work there instead. I was left under no illusion as to my future prospects in the hospital as the health department had been trying to shut it down for a long time.

Despite our meagre financial resources, we had decided, with the blessing of our head of department, to move emergency mountain medicine forward, as at that time there was no basic structure for its provision. The Big Chief, our Paris-trained anaesthetist and resuscitation specialist, was no stranger to the mountains. He and his brother had explored the entire Mont Blanc range from top to bottom during their stays in the family holiday chalet. Big Chief and his brother stood a full head taller than everybody else and they looked like a pair of spindly waders, especially Big Chief whose voice carried much further than anybody else's. Both brothers had a somewhat stately bearing, particularly Big Chief who was the elder of the two. I liked to imagine their younger selves tackling the greatest climbs in the range, without eating or drinking a drop and without exchanging a word.

If his brother was a famous mountain guide and talented rock climber, Big Chief was unquestionably in charge of the hospital. I had just joined when he took over. I didn't have altogether great memories of his predecessor but I didn't know what to make of Big Chief when he arrived. He seemed pretty impressive but perhaps we should have held on to Little Chief whose bearing was more of a Dr-Know-It-All, except with sticky palms and trembling hands. Things didn't get off to a good start, as the presentations were made while I was in the middle of trying to get an IV-line into a poor old woman who was so dehydrated and her veins so fragile we couldn't get her set up on a drip.

Getting an IV into a patient is a delicate manoeuvre that consists in finding a large vein that is not visible on the surface of the skin and introducing a catheter into it. There are several methods. The standard techniques require finding either the femoral vein at the top of the thigh or the subclavian vein, which as the name suggests is under the clavicle or collarbone. To do this, you insert a trocar, or tube, under the bone and follow specific points in an attempt to find the invisible vein and catheterize it. The first difficulty you encounter is finding the vein itself, then you have to introduce a metallic tube that looks like a bike gear cable into it, to guide the catheter into place, before removing it again. All that without losing your cool, shaking or perforating the artery of the same name that is lurking in the same place. All apprenticeships involve faltering first steps and it goes without saying that I had hit the subclavian artery and not the vein and was now applying swabs like a madman in a desperate attempt at damage limitation. Dr-Know-It-All was showing his successor round and introduced me with a dismissive gesture, spicing his comments with pathetic jokes, pleased to be able to put me down in front of an audience.

After an observation period of a few, mostly silent, months, Big Chief commenced his spring-cleaning campaign and wasn't content with just the obvious things. We had to face the fact the guy was good, really good, and was quite a character. He could also be irritating; in fact sometimes he was absolutely infuriating. His greatest pleasure in life was verbal jousting, an area in which he excelled, a bit like Jackie Chan leaving three adversaries rolling dazed on the floor at ten-metre intervals. I loved it, even if on occasion I was the one to come off worst. Not everybody was the same as me and over the years Big Chief made lots of friends but also a great deal of enemies.

Big Chief started off by appointing himself as the doctor responsible for mountain rescues, a role that was previously held by our surgeon. The latter was happy to relinquish the responsibility, recognizing that he would, as long as he lived, never ever climb aboard what he called 'that flying mountain-rescue cattle-truck'.

As for me, I had done my first rescue missions with the EMHM the year before joining the casualty department at the hospital. I remember as if it were yesterday my first contact with the rescue team. I turned up at the helipad for my first mission in my fire engine red Talbot van. The welcome at Les Bois Drop Zone was somewhat lukewarm to say the least. The elderly hang-glider attached to the top of my old banger didn't quite reflect the doctor's image. I slid down on to the battered old sofa in the common room of the small chalet that acted as an office, trying not to draw too much attention to myself. I nervously waited for the first call to come in, not knowing how or if my humble services were going to be required by the team. At this stage it was difficult to judge if I was considered an enemy or a fellow team member. Most of them were guides and I still had nothing to prove my skills as a mountaineer. The Tour de France was on the TV and the daily ritual, while waiting to be called out, was to watch the coverage, removing any opportunity I might have had of gleaning any kind of information about the job.

Among the older rescuers were those who had authority over the others and who took decisions, particularly about whether they needed to take a doctor on a mission or not. There was Jack, nicknamed the Professor, who had a way and manner of teaching rescue and resuscitation techniques with almost surgical precision. I listened with bemusement as he described the cardiac massage methods to me one by one, knowing full well that a heart will restart when it's good and ready, no matter what technique is used! Yet I always had a lot of respect for the old guys.

Then there was Douge, who was a bit gruff and for whom medicine was no more useful than parapsychology. Ironically, he was one of the first rescuers to accept me into the team and I have fond memories of the rescues we worked on together. Douge loved cycling and treasured his gleaming bike. One evening, while turning round to go home after being on call, my friend Jean-Bernard, also a doctor, had the misfortune to drive over it leaving the bike folded in half like a book. The Tour de France took one on the chin that night!

The dog-handler Yvan was quiet and efficient. Adja, the dog, was the complete opposite of Yvan: impulsive and difficult to control. Like all dogs restrained by training, he was continually on his guard, waiting, the price an avalanche dog has to pay. At the slightest whistle from a helicopter engine you would have to hold on tight to have any chance of stopping him leaping into action. Adja was straining, on the verge of an epileptic fit. The least sign from Yvan and he was off, exploding out of his starting blocks like an Olympic sprinter. And woe betide anyone who got in his way; his arrival in the cockpit was often a pretty violent affair.

At the end of evening memories of team members past and present were recalled. The rescuers were known among themselves as 'crampons'. 'Crampon' was usually put before the name with everyone free to substitute an attribute that best summed up a particular person. Crampon-foie-gras, for example, was the nickname of the man who every year would bring back the precious foodstuff from his native Périgord in order to do a bit of business on the side. Crampon-TV always talked to the news on the TV. And there were Crampon-tedious, Crampon-that-pisses-me-off and many others.

Crampon-danger-man was a mountain rescuer brought in from the Pyrénées Orientales. It was a miracle he was still alive. He had seen generations of young show-offs come through and knew a thing or two about it all. There was always someone pulling his leg, and to tease him a number of the gendarmes called him Crampon-pain-in-the-arse. You would be wise to stay out of his way if it looked like he didn't find it funny, as he was as strong as an ox and could hit like one too!

My first major rescue, of Bill the American, was with Crampon-danger-man. It's not easy to forget and is the story of a man snatched from the jaws of death.

DANGER-MAN

· · · · · · · · ·

It was a quiet summer's day at the end of the season. I was at a loose end and was enjoying carrying out a silly scientific experiment that involved attaching heart monitor patches to the chests of the pilot and Didier, his mechanic. The pilot's nickname was the Buzzard, and he will be long remembered in Chamonix. He didn't get his nickname from his looks, but from his flying technique. He had a very personal, and probably rather unconventional, way of handling the joystick that was nevertheless extremely effective. Some said that he must have been born with a joystick up his arse.

One day as we were returning to the base from Megève, I had asked him if he could land his Alouette helicopter like a jumbo jet. The Buzzard, who was something of a gambling man, took me at my word and started heading down the landing strip at 150 kilometres an hour, passing over it so close that I thought it was going to scratch the paintwork. The hangar seemed to be approaching us at breakneck speed and I asked myself where I thought he envisaged landing the craft. The moment came when we only had two options left: crash head-long into the hangar or take out a wall as we veered sideways, trying to hug the edge of the building. I have to admit I was a bit tense by this stage. I had started saying a few quick prayers when he had the bright idea of pulling violently on the joystick. We shot up into the air like the space shuttle *Columbia* before plunging back down to the left, throwing me against the bubble-shaped windscreen. Finally, the machine touched down as gently as an autumn leaf, smack-bang on the landing spot, without the slightest tremor, and with a mocking smile playing across the pilot's lips.

It was with the Buzzard, Didier the mechanic, Crampon-danger-man and another rescuer nicknamed Fred that I took off late that afternoon for a routine mission to the Glacier des Améthystes. We were supposed to pick up an old aircraft engine that the glacier had spat out, doubtless after several long years of digestion. It was probably from an old crate that had crashed in a storm during the Second World War. The engine had resurfaced and we had to winch it down to Chamonix. It was a code WEUWAC (will end up with a collector) clean-up operation.

The engine was heavier than it looked and handling it was a more delicate process than we had imagined, so the crew was deep in concentration.

'Bravo Lima, this is Cordial. Take a look at the south face of the Droites. A guy's had a fall.'

Bravo Lima was the blue gendarmerie helicopter's codename and Cordial was the Chamonix mountain rescue headquarters, which at that time was based in the Place du Mont Blanc.

We left the engine where it was and went to have a look. The change in programme filled me with a mixture of nerves and excitement. At last, this looked like a real emergency and a real rescue!

After whirling round the Argentière basin for a few moments we dropped on to the south side of the impressive mountain that is the Droites. I had climbed it once via the most direct line, known as the Ginat Route, in winter with Teddy, a beefy bloke from the Groupe militaire de haute montagne (GMHM). It has a magnificent vertical 1,000-metre wall of ice that is as cold as its gloomy face suggests. It should appear on any mountaineer's list of great climbs. We started up the route at around midday with the idea of making a nocturnal ascent. This was thanks to my slightly absurd pet principle that you didn't bivouac in winter, the best tactic being to climb at night. That way, if you take too long the worst that can happen is you get caught out in daylight. So Teddy and I had spent the night on the route, descending via the same couloir that the five of us were now scrutinizing, looking for the slightest clue.

It was the end of the summer, the sun was melting the snow on the mountain's south face and mudslides regularly joined the cone of debris beneath it. We hovered over the foot of the funnel until we finally spotted a shape that could be human, half-buried under a pile of rocks.

The final rappel anchor must have failed. Rocks were continuing to pour down the runnel. It looked like the bloke was toast to me, unless he was made of toughened steel. The Buzzard gently brought us closer in to make sure it was our guy. We were only a few metres from the pillar next to the cone of debris and could sense the whole mountain was unstable. There was a real risk that the draught from the machine's rotor blades would dislodge blocks at any moment. It was our man all right, we could see the colour of his jacket now, which must have been yellow before being dragged through the gravel-filled slush and snow.

'There he is! Down there!' shouted Fred, thinking he had spotted him first.

'Yeah, but it's not looking good,' replied Danger-man, 'with all the stuff that's fallen on top of him.'

It seemed clear to us that there wasn't much we could do. It was the victim's climbing partner who had walked to the Couvercle hut to call for help. I made a quick calculation in my head about how long the climber had been there, knowing that it takes a good hour to walk to the hut.

The Buzzard circled round to get a better view of the terrain and the state of our poor bloke below. We came in again, and something incredible happened: to our amazement, our supposed cadaver moved one of its arms.

The first comment in the helicopter was:

'Shit, he's alive!'

'Unbelievable,' Didier added helpfully.

We were all wondering how this man had survived such a huge fall and avalanche of rock. It reminded me of the acromegalic killer from the James Bond movies who was built like a tank and had steel teeth. It didn't matter if his car had landed at the bottom of a ravine, he'd been thrown from a train or several tonnes of scaffolding had collapsed on top of him, he would always come out of it unscathed.

It was impossible for us to treat the victim safely where he was so Danger-man decided to set Fred and me down on a patch of snow a little lower down to lighten the helicopter. He would then pick up the climber and pull him out of the oversized bowling alley. This technique is known as the 'sling' and allows us to extract the victim from the danger zone as quickly as we can, while exposing the team to the least amount of risk.

A rescuer is winched down as close as possible to the victim. The rescuer clips a separate rope to the victim's harness and is then winched back into the helicopter, which moves away from the rock as soon as it can. The victim is hoisted up on the end of the rope, suspended in mid-air, before being set down in a safer place. This certainly isn't the best way to transport an injured person but sometimes there's no other choice.

I remember seeing our man, who was called Bill, suspended, motionless like a sack of potatoes, from the rope attached to his belly, turning round and round in the light of the setting sun. His arms and legs dangled like those of some double-jointed marionette. I preferred not to think about the state of his spine.

The helicopter deposited him into our arms, completely dis-located, like some kind of offering. I felt his bones crack and splinter under my hands, as if the slightest movement on our part would finish him off.

'I'll prepare the stretcher,' said Fred.

The victim was worryingly still and there wasn't the slight-est groan or whimper coming from him. He had given up, as if he had summoned up his last ounce of strength to move his arm as we flew over and had nothing else left. At first I thought the winching had killed him, then, looking closer, I saw that he was still breathing, but it was very shallow.

'He's still alive! I'll get an IV-line in him and let's get out of here. Tell the helicopter I need five minutes ...'

The helicopter flew off into the Argentière basin to let us work in peace. I don't remember what I did or didn't do right, but he had oxygen and was on a drip that was re-expanding his veins and giving him a chance to hang on. I was a beginner and was still learning, no one could have asked any more from me. What else dare I try? The Buzzard picked us up and dived like a bird of prey down towards the Leschaux glacier, skimming the roof of the hut of the same name before dropping like a bomb down the Gorges de l'Arveyron. We whirled over jagged blades of gleaming ice and I can still hear the thump of the rotor blades. In a few minutes we were ready to land, the famous request of 'landing DZ', that we heard fifteen times a day over the radio, had been given. At that time Chamonix hospital was still housed in a building on the road out of town towards Les Praz. We couldn't land on the roof and would set down at the Clos de Savoie or the ice rink instead. A half-tonne of steel straining to land flat on its belly on tarmac without crashing is always a magical and irrationally exciting moment.

Despite only being able to give Bill a meagre amount of medical assistance, I wasn't too displeased with myself. I had got his blood pressure up a bit and hadn't wasted too much time bringing him down. My heart was racing and his had held on.

Once the helicopter had landed we were still 100 metres from the hospital. We also had a road to cross and needed the help of the firemen. We took the wounded man out of the helicopter and loaded him into the red fire service ambulance, only to unload him again five minutes later at the accident and emergency unit. The only dispensation we got was to drive the wrong way down the road, rather than having to drive all the way round the town's one-way system.

None of this was of much help to Bill who was slowly starting to slip away.

The Chamonix hospital, at that time, was something else. It was an old hotel that over the years had been converted section by section, room by room, and was a hospital in name and function only.

We deposited Bill in the only place that bore any resemblance to a resuscitation area, a stretcher in one of the wretched rooms that made up our modest A&E department.

We had hardly finished unloading Bill when he went into cardiac arrest. This hardly surprised me, given the state he was in when we found him, the amount of blows to the head he had sustained and the manner in which we winched him off the mountain. Bill would have stayed in cardiac arrest if it hadn't been for Big Chief. Rigorous in his habits, Big Chief handled the situation with all the authority and skill for which he was known. Bill's heart was beating again and his blood pressure had improved, after a fashion. With a breathing tube up his nose and a few well-chosen cardiac drugs in his system, Bill was back with us.

At the same time, we did as many x-rays as we could manage without moving him around too much. His list of injuries was a long one. If memory serves me right, which isn't the case and I must have forgotten some things, he had thirty-two fractures, including both femurs, his pelvis, at least ten ribs, his right humerus, open fractures to both wrists, his back was broken in three different places and naturally he had a fractured skull too. This doesn't include the secondary breaks, a number of which were also open. To top it all, the scan we had given him with the hospital's one ultrasound machine showed the presence of a retroperitoneal haematoma. This meant he had internal bleeding, which didn't make his prognosis any better.

Bill was transferred to Geneva's cantonal hospital. That was the end of the story and we heard no more from him for five years. Then one day, the telephone rang on the reception desk at the new PGHM building near the church.

'Hello. Excuse me, sorry, is that the Chamonix mountain rescue service?' a voice asked in French with an American accent.

'Yes, this is the Chamonix PGHM,' replied the man on duty.

'I ... fell on the Droites, five years ago ... I had a rescue ... I want to know the name of the rescuers ... Is it possible?'

'It's possible but I'll have to check the records.'

That same evening I got a call from Danger-man.

'Hey, Manu, can you come down?'

'Hi, Henry, it's been a while.'

'Do you remember Bill the American?'

'Er, no ... Unless you mean ... Not our guy from the Droites?'

'Yeah, that's the one, and he's here!'

'What d'you mean, here?'

'In Chamonix, stupid. He wants to take us out to dinner this evening, at the Peter Pan.'

Sitting back in my chair, pleasantly full after my plate of beef with morel mushrooms and potatoes au gratin, I sipped my fourth glass of expensive red wine. I was slightly dazed after our hearty meal and watched the man who had made such a miraculous recovery. Bill was having a great time and he was so pleased to see us. There he was, sitting in front of us and not even in a wheelchair. Of course, he was covered in scars and his head was a slightly funny shape but he was there having fun, with his wife gazing adoringly at him. Three months in a coma, thirteen operations and four years of physiotherapy must have blown a hole in his health insurance, but he had refused to give up.

I couldn't get over it.

2

WINTER

BLUE CATHEDRAL

• • • • • • • • •

I had been doing the job for fifteen years. A decade and a half of mountain rescues in the Mont Blanc range, an extraordinary mountain arena twenty kilometres long by ten kilometres wide, an incredible playground bristling with peaks of rock and ice where, as at sea, conditions can change from one second to the next. When I was a young arrogant idiot I thought I had pretty much seen and done it all. As I grew older and wiser and the first grey hairs started to appear, my memory filled with moments of great happiness with good friends, friends whom I would see die horrifically in front of me a few days later. I'll never understand what it is that draws us to such a strange and perverse place. Beauty, a sense of space, the effort involved, the danger … a reason for living?

It was the start of the week, one January. There had been a huge fall of snow two weeks before. A high-pressure weather system had set in and it didn't seem to want to leave. I was ready for my umpteenth winter season: my pack had been dusted off and the out-of-date vials had been replaced, but I still needed a new pair of gloves as mine were wrecked.

What were they going to fall down this year? Which friend was I going to have to pick up? And what was I going to get wrong? Why was I experiencing such a mixture of feelings about it all? Sometimes I was on one side of the line and other times I was on the other ... I spent so much time finding the traps that other people fell into, but was I really immune from them myself?

Six-thirty a.m. The phone in the hospital staff room was making a commotion. I didn't like the sound of it: too often it meant trouble was heading our way. Thankfully the night had been quiet and I hadn't been disturbed by too many 'Doctor, I've got sunburn and it hurts' or by drunken Swedes injured in fights taking it out on me because I had to stitch them up. There was only the low din of the hospital's central heating boiler, which was under the staff dorm, to get on my nerves. It was like spending the night in an Airbus.

I was in a daze. Virginie, the nurse who started at six-thirty on the morning shift, woke me up. She spoke quietly. She knew I didn't like commotion in the mornings.

'Manu, get dressed. The PGHM guys are coming to get you for a crevasse rescue.'

'Yeah ... Already? What time is it?'

'Six-thirty ... Rise and shine, doc.'

Someone in a crevasse at six in the morning in the middle of winter, what was going on? Nine times out of ten, accidents in crevasses at this time of year are on the Vallée Blanche but they usually happen at around midday. That's picnic time, when it's a bit warmer and people are starting to relax. When skiers of all shapes and sizes, nationalities and political persuasions, converge on the Géant icefall, jostling their way through a narrow section of snow-covered séracs. A wander around the place in summer gives you an idea of the state of the glacier: it's got more holes than a Swiss cheese.

I had to get dressed. Underpants, red Gore-Tex. A quick hello in the A&E corridor on the way out. My harness with its sturdy screw-link from the ironmongers for winching, my boots and, if possible, the crampons that went with them.

The classic mistake was to change boots before going back on duty and forgetting to adjust your crampons. It had happened to me when I was starting out. The rescue was on the north face of the Tour Ronde, which is well known for the poor quality of the ice, especially in the middle section. It is still described in some guidebooks as a summer route, which fails to take account of the fact that the snow conditions aren't what they used to be. It was as I was trying to get the blasted crampons on, doubled up in the only two spare metres of room in the back of the helicopter, that I realised my mistake. They were one stop too short to fit over my boots. I didn't dare say anything and strapped them on to my feet as best I could, hoping they would hold. As I reached the stance where the two other rescuers were already clipped in and my feet came into contact with the ice, I heard a sinister metal clanging. My crampons had fallen off and were dangling from their straps. It is a dreaded noise that will throw a climber off balance in the twinkling of an eye. I just gave my colleagues a sheepish look. Luckily, the victim who had fallen had ended up level with the belay, which the two rescuers had strengthened by adding a couple of ice screws. This meant I didn't have to use my crampons. They had a good laugh at my expense for the rest of the day. It is perhaps thanks to this incident that they now call us 'Crampon-Docs'.

There was no time for daydreaming that morning, the helicopter was already there. Today it was the red helicopter, Dragon 74, used by the Sécurité Civile (civil defence or security authorities) and not the Sécurité Sociale (social security), as my son called it! At the joystick was Gérard and he was ably assisted by Xav, his scrupulous mechanic. Gérard loved to explain things and thanks to him I knew about virtually all the buttons and screens on the instrument panel. With a bit of luck, but only if it was really necessary, I might be able to land one of the things on my own.

'What's the problem?' I asked.

'We got a call from a guide. His client's fallen into a crevasse by the Helbronner. We've got no idea how he is ...'

'Ah,' I managed to reply, still half asleep. I thought how nice it would have been to start the day with a cup of good strong coffee.

I sat down in the corner, at the back of the helicopter, in a daydream contemplating the succession of sharp peaks rushing before my eyes. There's nothing to beat the flight up the Vallée Blanche early in the morning, even if you have seen it a hundred times before.

We came in low next to the Col d'Entrèves and the site of the accident. The altimeter must have been touching 3,000 metres. Through the windows we could make out a small group of people and a tiny black hole. There was the glorious sight of the sun peeping through the Flambeaux. It was right in front of us and at that moment, without a thought for the horror that possibly awaited me down the crevasse, I thought what a great job I had.

Then it was kicking-out time, into the cold and the din, the opening of the sliding door my cue to leave the warmth and comfort of the cabin. It was so nice in there … We picked up the extra gear – snow stakes, static rope and a few bags – we needed for the rescue. Then there was the usual racket of the helicopter flying off and we were rewarded with a huge gust of wind and faces full of snow. All this was enough to wake me up.

Silence. When the helicopter flies away the contrast is huge and the quiet of the mountains takes over again.

The rescue team was already in action. I found them surprisingly relaxed for an accident in a crevasse, the looks on their faces immediately putting me at ease. It didn't look like it was that bad after all.

There was Marcel Benzalès, always in a good mood, with his Salvador Dalí moustache. The one drawback with Marcel was his slightly jumpy avalanche rescue dog, Jimmy. The creature had already gone for more than one of us. My mate Barnab was also there, and the dismayed look on his face when he saw me coming could be translated as 'Oh no, not him'. Then I recognized the guide who had raised the alarm: it was Whitey. He was my hero. He was well into his fifties and just as active as ever. His hair was the same colour as his beard, grey-white all over. He was a jack-of-all-trades – master carpenter, joiner, plumber – and he was always on the go, up early in the morning walking in the mountains. The guy never stopped.

This time things were not going well, at least not for his client. He greeted me as enthusiastically as ever, which reassured me. If he was relaxed it meant his client was ok. And I knew what it was like to lose a client down a crevasse. In fact, I wondered which guide hadn't seen the same thing. The club seemed to be growing just lately.

Whitey was squinting in the cold.

'Hi, Manu, have you seen the hole?'

'Yeah, I saw. Is it deep?'

'Forty metres …'

'And it's your client at the bottom of it?'

'Yes, but he's ok. It's incredible. He gave me a scare. I thought he was dead.'

I clipped myself to the safety rope the other rescuers had set up and moved over to say hello. They were deep in concentration, setting up the winch and static rope. There was quite a relaxed atmosphere for though the situation was pretty serious, they made it look like they did this kind of thing every day.

One of the rescuers, Hervé, was already in the crevasse. Given the height of the fall, he wasn't convinced the guy was ok. We try to teach rescuers to be on their guard with victims of falls into crevasses. They are often much more badly injured than is first apparent. The cold has an anaesthetic effect and claustrophobia makes them want to get out of the hole as soon as possible. The victims seem to forget that they are badly injured, and experience has shown that the seriousness of their internal injuries is often underestimated. The policy of doctors first on the scene is to assume that the victims have multiple injuries. We have all been caught out at one time or another by someone with a broken neck we didn't spot or an undiagnosed ruptured spleen.

Nowadays, we are so conscientious it is almost comical. Half the time we pick up people who aren't badly injured at all. The second they are out of the crevasse we lie them flat, strap them to the stretcher, get them on oxygen and before they can speak they are being whisked away by helicopter. Ten minutes later the nurses and nursing auxiliaries are rushing to strip the clothes from them, as the medical textbooks state that 'any victim with suspected multiple injuries must be completely undressed and correctly examined'. Two hours later, not having found any juicy symptoms we can get our teeth into, we politely ask them to leave the examination room so that we can usher the next patient in. We then see them standing in their socks by the payphone in the hall holding a bin bag full of their wet or torn clothing. They are trying to call their friends to come and pick them up. But they of course are still in the mountains with the car keys in their pockets …

'Manu, you go down and make sure he hasn't broken anything and tell us what you need to bring him up,' ordered Marcel.

'Yep.'

I get really excited going down into crevasses and I love doing medicine in dangerous situations. Ironically, that's when I do some of my best doctoring. The blue world forty metres inside the ice is a special place where, for once, I can make my own decisions. There are no eminent physicians looking over my shoulder, pestering me and telling me what to do. It is an unusual environment, but it's one where I feel at home.

The cold, the water running down your neck, the snow intent on burying the victim as quickly as you can uncover him or her, all make administering emergency care to a patient under these circumstances far from simple. The patient, if he or she doesn't look dead, will more often than not be freezing cold and very agitated.

You have two options. The first involves giving them a shot and going through the complicated process of anaesthetizing them to put them to sleep and relieve the pain. However, a crevasse is hardly the best place for this kind of delicate procedure. Trying to find a minuscule vein that's more often than not gone into spasm because of the cold and the effects of hypotension and is hidden under layers of clothes, can be a rather tricky operation. Then there are the technical aspects and side-effects of the drugs. Winching is an equally complicated manoeuvre, as bringing up a stretcher with all the equipment needed for critical care, including an oxygen bottle, is no mean feat. It is just asking the tubes to come undone, leaving the patient no longer hooked up to the respirator, the perfect moment for him or her to go into cardiac arrest.

This method is great every time it works, but it can also very quickly turn into a complete nightmare taking up to anything over an hour to get right.

The other option is the vet method. I have turned to it at various times down the years, even if it has been frowned upon for a long time by those who, it goes without saying, have never worked under these conditions. A good intramuscular injection of Ketamine through the trousers and straight into the arse will put anyone to sleep in less than three minutes. The patient's body becomes rigid but he or she is still breathing, which means you don't have to take all the usual ironmongery into the crevasse.

The effects of Ketamine have been well known since the Vietnam war when it was heavily used. It causes a trance-like state, a bit like catalepsy, characterized by a fixed stare, the muscles tensing up and decreased sensitivity to pain. It keeps the blood pressure up, and the muscular rigidity provides a natural splint for any broken bones. Moreover, it doesn't affect the body's involuntary breathing mechanism, which means the doctor doesn't have to carry out a tracheal intubation and place the patient on a mechanical respirator.

Once the patient is on the surface and more comfortable, it is good practice to give him or her oxygen and a sedative. Without this, Ketamine has the annoying habit of bringing on severe and unpleasant hallucinations.

Only a few dozen years ago victims were hauled up to the surface, irrespective of their injuries. They would be pulled up by whatever came to hand, a harness, jacket or even a leg. The tools used at that time were quite often ingenious homemade affairs that wouldn't have looked out of place in a torture chamber. Although this method has the advantage of being a particularly quick solution, it is rarely used these days as, even if the victim is not badly injured, the consequences of such a rescue can be more serious than one might think. And it hurts.

A colleague of mine at a conference a few years ago mentioned a little-known condition with a rather unwieldy name. Bezold Jarisch syndrome is where a victim left hanging for too long in his or her harness can go into cardio-respiratory arrest brought about by compression of the femoral artery and the heart being deprived of blood. This means that care strategies have to be modified accordingly. Taking all these considerations into account, we have to go into the crevasses.

While I put my crampons on, Whitey explained what had happened. He and his client had set out to do the north face of the Tour Ronde. They slept in the Torino hut, on the Italian side of Mont Blanc, to get a dawn start. It was a perfectly understandable decision, as even though the route can be done in a day, Hubert, who worked as a notary, wasn't a very fast climber. A good early start could only improve their chances of success. They happily headed out one behind the other with climbing skins on their skis, traversing below the north face of the Col d'Entrèves, the most logical approach route.

They rounded the first rocky outcrop and picked up an old set of ski tracks that was windswept but still visible. They came to a dubious depression in the snow barring their route. Whitey, who knew what he was looking for, spotted it immediately. The depression wasn't very wide, a ski length at the most. Plus, the snow was cold, settled and firm, suggesting there would be no problem with it. Whitey crossed it at right angles, reducing the risk of falling in, and carried on. Hubert cheerfully followed behind him, completely unaware.

Suddenly, he stopped stock-still. A chasm had opened up underneath him. Only the tips of his skis were resting on the edge of the hole in front, while the backs of his skis sat on the lip behind him. Under his feet were forty metres of nothing. The snowbridge, which had held under the weight of Whitey, had collapsed with a dull thud as Hubert crossed it.

Terrified the rest of the snowbridge would fall in underneath him, Hubert didn't dare shout out and instead let out a muffled whimper. This brought Whitey, who had calmly gone on ahead unaware of the problem, out of his reverie. He turned around.

'Whatever you do, don't move!' he screamed.

If there was one thing Hubert didn't fancy doing at that moment, it was moving.

Whitey got as close as he could and quickly took off his skis to make an anchor. The next minute the rope was out of his bag. He tied a knot, clipped in a karabiner and the rope landed twenty centimetres from Hubert's skis. All he had to do was pick it up. But that meant bending down …

He clumsily put out a trembling hand. The snow held. He caught the karabiner. The snow was still holding. Then Hubert made a tiny unnecessary movement, shifting his weight slightly. The snow gave way. Hubert disappeared into the hole.

Whitey tensed his muscles like he was some kind of human crossbow to hold the rope. The shock was violent and the anchor held but it burnt.

'Hubert, it's ok. I've got you!' he yelled.

'I hadn't realized the danger he was in, I thought he was hanging from his harness,' he explained to me as I fastened my crampons.

'He was saying, "I'm going to die, I'm going to let go!" I told him it was ok, that I had him. I asked him how deep the crevasse was. He said 100 metres. I told him there weren't any 100 metre crevasses in Chamonix. He kept saying he was going to fall, that he was going to die. Then all of a sudden the rope went slack. I realized he hadn't had time to clip the karabiner to his harness. He was weighed down by his pack and skis and was only holding on to the karabiner. He finally just let go!'

Just thinking about it made the hairs on the back of my neck stand on end. I understood how terrified he must have been! I started my descent down into the depths of the crevasse where Hervé was waiting for me. I was suspended over nothingness from the end of a cable with a static rope as a back up. I entered a cathedral with glassy blue walls, its vaulted nave forty metres high. Everything looked tiny at the bottom. I was used to the environment, but nervous all the same.

Hubert was lying flat, trapped between the walls of ice that narrowed below. He had fallen on to a layer of snow created by the bridge when it collapsed. If he had fallen in further with it, he would probably have been dashed to pieces on the blocks of ice that carpeted the bottom of the crevasse.

'You ok, Hubert?'

'Yeah, I'm ok but I don't dare move,' he replied, having got over the initial shock.

Hervé gave me a worried look, although he was glad he had got me down. I started examining the patient as I always do: feeling first the head, then the neck, slight pressure to the sternum, two hands on the thorax. It's generally at this moment that the patient leaps up as I press a broken rib. Next I checked his belly. When it is distended and painful you can't rule out internal haemorrhaging, which is almost certainly caused by a ruptured spleen. What they don't write in the books is that the abdomen is often hard and distended in victims of hypothermia, without any internal haemorrhaging. Useful to know … After the belly, the pelvis. It is often injured during a fall in a crevasse, owing to the victim being wedged between narrowing walls of ice. We also check the legs, paying particular attention to how sensitive they are and how well the patient can move them. It's often extremely difficult to evaluate the state of the spine in the bottom of a crevasse. It is essential that we ascertain there is no latent tetraplegia or paraplegia, taking all necessary precautions.

'Right, what do we do now?' asked a slightly impatient Hervé, who had had enough of being in the gloomy crevasse.

'Shall I get the stretcher down here? Or the KED? Or both?'

I checked Hubert all over and he didn't seem to have any worrying symptoms. He was very sensible and wasn't moving, patiently waiting for us to tell him what to do. There didn't even seem much point in getting a catheter into him as he wasn't in any pain.

In the end we decided to pull him up in a KED, a brace used by a number of rescuers. It allows you to support and protect the victim's back along its entire length and is the ideal tool for giving your patient maximum protection when you can't use a stretcher.

Hubert was ready to be taken up to the surface. We obviously had to sort out the ropes a bit. With both the cable and static line, we were bound to get tangled up. But rescuers are masters of these kinds of manoeuvres. When a simple accident in a crevasse doesn't require too much medical input, they can have you out in under an hour. I don't think there are many better places in the world for it to happen.

I was dangling from the cable with Hubert and all of a sudden it felt very fragile indeed. I could feel the vibrations from the winch's motor through the slings holding me as it strained to bring us up. We finally popped out. The tricky part is not getting caught under the lip overhanging the top of the hole.

A great breath of fresh air awaited us on the surface. The sun warmed and dazzled us as if we had come out of a long tunnel. Hervé came up after us with all the equipment. The tension dissipated. This rescue had been technical but had gone well and there had been no injuries. Hubert was happy, perhaps even happier than if he had climbed the route.

THE SLENDER THREAD

· · · · · · · · ·

'Slow down, Rémi! Your steps are too big!'

Catherine was a bit annoyed that morning. Rémi had launched himself at the climb with gusto. He sometimes tended to forget that his legs were twice as long as Catherine's. She preferred to start gently, warm up a bit and set her own pace. She had strong calves and could stay the distance.

Good-looking with clear blue eyes, Rémi was always keen to help. His main asset was his size. And it was his main drawback too, as everything about him was big, including his hands. He was no fan of 7c climbs. While his mates could pull up on a tiny crimp, he could only get the flesh of one fingertip over it. He sometimes almost daydreamed about getting frostbite to shorten his fingers. In any case, he didn't get his mountain guide's badge for his rock climbing. It was thanks to his skills as an all-rounder. He was particularly at ease on steep slopes of rotten ice. He could run face first down slopes that others would battle their way down on all fours. In fact, Rémi was a bit of an intellectual. He had never worked as a mountain guide, but had completed the training out of a sense of duty to his father and brother, both professional guides. He earned his living as an engineer specializing in motorway construction, and mountaineering was his escape. It was as if by going into the mountains he was making amends for the violence he was inflicting on the environment in the course of his job. It was a kind of penance.

That winter Rémi had decided to do the Contamine-Grisolle on the Mont Blanc du Tacul. The route wasn't in very good condition but that didn't bother him as he liked that kind of climbing. They had left the hut very early that morning as they were expected back in Grenoble that evening, to collect their children who were staying with Catherine's mother.

'Slack, Catherine. It's not hard, just pay out the rope.'

'Hang on, Rémi, it's caught.'

Catherine tried to unravel the tangle of knots at her feet. The feeble light from her headtorch didn't help very much. To top it all, she had a cold and couldn't stop sniffing, it was miserable.

'Give me some slack, I'm still climbing.'

'I said hang on a moment, it's all knotted up!' snapped Catherine.

'Right, well, I'll put an ice screw in.'

Catherine could hear Rémi grumbling to himself.

Suddenly a volley of plates of ice came crashing down. A bit the size of a pizza dish shattered as it hit her left hand. Even with gloves on, it really hurt.

'Careful, Rémi, you're chucking ice all over me!'

'Mind out the way …'

'Thanks, it's a bit late now.'

Catherine tried moving her aching hand. Luckily there was nothing broken.

Rémi had started on the bergschrund above and the ice was pretty rotten. With each blow of his ice axes he sent shards of ice everywhere. It's not hard, he told himself, just a bit dicey…

bugger. He pulled off the first Charlet Moser ice screw that came to hand on his harness and screwed it in two centimetres. All of a sudden the entire plate of ice came away and took the ice screw with it. Shit, there goes a brand new Charlet Moser. What an idiot. Never mind, we'll have to do without, Rémi said to himself. He carried on climbing, swearing as his front points skidded on the ice.

Two hours later dawn was breaking. Catherine was pleased with herself, as she had managed to pick up the ice screw Rémi had dropped. That'll cost him a beer, she thought. Rémi had changed route, as it was quite warm for 3,600 metres. The narrow section over granite above the first ice slope didn't look very attractive and two stones had already fallen down from it. Rémi heard them whistle past his ears before ricocheting down the ice. Even if it wasn't the normal route, the left-hand option, which consisted in turning the shoulder by the snowy couloir to the side, seemed safer. He was disappointed by the poor quality of the ice. Studying the face from the hut the evening before, it had looked like there was firm snow in this section. In reality it was powder: an unstable thin layer of snow covering crappy grey ice.

His calves screaming, Rémi continued to lead whole pitches without putting in a single ice screw. Each time he thought about putting in some gear, he dismissed the idea, telling himself the ice might be better higher up. His philosophy was that if you place gear it has to hold. Here, on this kind of ground ice screws wouldn't hold.

Ten minutes later Catherine heard the sound of another climber's ice axes. He or she had obviously chosen the same line as them. She didn't really like this kind of climbing, it made her nervous. She had had to pull herself together more than once to get the blasted ice axe in. She was getting tired. Luckily, she was climbing up diagonally, otherwise the lumps of ice she was sending down would have already decapitated the bloke climbing below.

'Hi!' said the other climber as he came up alongside her.

'Hi.'

Catherine was having a rest. She wanted to stretch out her ankle as she held on to the ice axe, but she couldn't find a comfortable position.

'I'm Bernie.'

'Er, Catherine,' came the strained reply.

She found him a little forward in the introductions and she was a little bit miffed about being overtaken so easily.

'Great, isn't it?'

'Erm, not really. The ice is no good.'

At that precise moment in time, Catherine couldn't give a damn about the views. The one thing on her mind was the amount of climbing they had to reach the shoulder of the Tacul. It seemed never-ending.

'Yeah, but we can't complain. It could be worse.'

He was soloing the whole thing. He looked young, probably a local who spent every morning doing this kind of thing.

He set off again. But she couldn't help noticing that he didn't look all that comfortable. It looked to her as if he was making a show of speeding up a bit. As he passed above her he sent a lump of ice hurtling down to her right. She let out a little cry, not because it had hit her but to let him know that she was below him.

'Sorry. I'll go left, so I don't knock ice down on you.'

'Now there's an idea,' muttered Catherine.

The idea of the climber soloing above her hardly put her mind at rest. She had never seen the attraction of something that she thought was completely daft. It was bad enough she was roped up to someone else on a slope of sheet ice. All of a sudden she missed her children.

The shoulder of the Tacul was only about 200 metres away. Catherine started to get bad cramp in her calves. The sun had risen to the east of the massif and toyed with the buttresses on the Dent du Géant, before its warm fingers caressed the ice face.

The solo climber had now gone left of Rémi and was making his way up the final pitches of glassy ice. He seemed to be going too fast for such a long route. His line made a perfect arc coming back right, as the cornice straight above blocked access to the shoulder. He was now right above Rémi. He still seemed to be setting quite a pace, but something told the climbers below that he would soon start to show signs of fatigue.

A few minutes later Rémi found a kind of depression where the ice seemed good enough to set up a belay stance, so that he could rest his calf muscles and belay Catherine properly. She had completely lost her footing twice already. He placed two ice screws, which meant he could clip himself to something for the first time on the whole route.

'On belay, Catherine, I've got you. The ice is gr ...'

He was in mid-sentence when a sound of shattering glass rang out above him. He felt his blood run cold and he clung instinctively to the ice, not moving. He watched as a lump of ice the size of a small table fell past his left side. It spun and ricocheted down the slope, its shattered fragments disappearing among the séracs hanging over the exit from the Pointe Lachenal. Rémi expected to see their soloist fall down after the shards of ice. But no, reassuringly he was still above Rémi's head, even if he had sent down a huge block.

Rémi felt himself getting tense. The lump of ice had really put the wind up him and the other climber was getting on his nerves. The ice was bad enough, he didn't need anyone else making him more nervous. The other bloke could play silly buggers somewhere else, as far as Rémi was concerned.

He carefully lifted up his head to see what the soloist was up to. It looked like there was a problem, he was trying to get an ice screw in and clip himself to it while he pawed fruitlessly at the ice with his right foot.

'Oi! You ok?' shouted Rémi.

'Er …'

'And be careful with all that ice, that last bit almost hit us.'

'Sorry.'

Rémi carried on bringing Catherine up.

'Hey! I've broken my crampon,' the other climber finally shouted out.

Rémi looked up and saw that one of his feet wasn't attached to the ice. He must have lost the front part. That kind of thing didn't happen with rigid crampons whose two sections are firmly bolted together. The guy hadn't even thought to use proper equipment. He had placed his ice axes as best he could, clipping himself to one of them, and was trying to find a solution to his predicament. In short, he didn't look at all comfortable.

'Hey, I'm really screwed. I think I'm going to have to cut steps.'

'Don't talk nonsense. Cutting steps in 100 metres of ice, with us underneath. You've got to be joking!'

Rémi didn't like the sound of this. Not one little bit. Plus, it was they who were going to get faces full of ice. No way. He had to sort out something else.

'Hang on,' he shouted. 'Wait for me to get to you and I'll put you on a rope for the final section.'

'That's kind, thanks. But I think I'll be ok. Don't worry about it.'

Quite the contrary, Rémi was now extremely worried. The guy might be ballsy but he was just out of school, still a teen-ager. Rémi had absolutely no confidence in his ability to get out of this on his own. The plates of ice were going to fall straight on to their heads and him with them. It was out of the question.

'I said hang on. I'm coming!' yelled Rémi, as he got ready to set off.

'It's ok, I'm fine,' replied Bernie.

He was trying as best he could to scrape out steps for his feet, but his cramponless boot barely scratched the surface of the ice. At that rate it was going to take him three days. Cath-erine, who had just got to the stance, was starting to panic.

'Do something, Rémi! He's going to fall and take us with him!'

Rémi took his mobile out of his pocket, swearing.

'I'm calling the helicopter. The guy's a complete idiot!'

The incident in the crevasse had made us hungry. Back at the Drop Zone, the DZ, a little breakfast was in order. The atmos-phere was relaxed. Tony was putting away the gear we had just used and checking the vacuum splints and the shell, a body vacuum mattress. We hadn't looked very clever the day before when unloading the guy with a supposed broken back. In the time it had taken us to transport him to the hospital, the shell had completely deflated. It must surely have a hole in it. The problem with gear is that you have to be sure at all times that it is in perfect working order for when it's needed. You have to be totally rigorous. While Tony was checking everything, I helped myself to a leftover croissant and a lukewarm coffee with the helicopter pilot Gérard and Xav, the mechanic.

It was a short break. Ten minutes later we were flying past the flanks of the Aiguille du Midi, propelled along by the first thermals of the day. Gérard had chosen to come this way to get to the Col du Midi. It always amazes me to look down on the superb routes on the Aiguille's north face. There's the Frendo, the Mallory, the Eugster and the Carli-Chassagne, routes over 1,000 metres long that I climbed when I first started mountaineering. It's incredible how easy they look when you fly over them in a helicopter. It makes you want to do them again, at a sprint.

The reassuring bulk of the Col du Midi appeared before us at 3,530 metres, immense and white. That was where the problem was.

'There! At eleven o'clock,' shouted Tony.

'Eleven o'clock … You sure?' said Gérard.

'Yeah, a little bit lower down, about 100 metres under the cornice.'

'Got it!'

As if to contradict what he had just said, Gérard headed off right, in the opposite direction.

'No, go left! Down there!' insisted Tony.

'Yeah, ok, calm down. I saw them. Let me see what's going on … I've got to go round. I want to see how we can come in. There's a lot of turbulence around here, especially if it's blowing in off Lake Geneva.'

Gérard knew the range too well to be caught out here, whereas we rescuers always just want to get to the victim as quickly as possible. The call Cordial had received had been a bit panicked, but you have to be careful as there is sometimes good reason to be alarmed. A man had called on his mobile, from his belay, to say that a solo climber was just inches away from peeling off the ice and wiping out several hundred metres below. What's more, he was going to fall on their heads … It looked like the rescue was going to be a bit tricky. We couldn't afford to make any mistakes.

Gérard rounded the shoulder of the Tacul. The conditions were safe and there didn't seem to be any obvious gusts of wind.

'Right, how are you going to do this, Tony?' asked Gérard.

Tony looked at the three mountaineers, specks in the middle of the immense 500-metre face. He weighed up the advantages and disadvantages of the various options. He had spent the last three months doing nothing but easy rescues, mainly reconnaissance flights, and now all of a sudden he was being asked to make *the* right decision. The stakes were pretty high.

'You'll have to get in a bit closer. I want to check which one we're going to pick up,' replied Tony.

The solo climber was the one above. He was absolutely terrified and looked like he could let go at any moment. The ice was black and glassy. The guy below had put his arms above his head asking for help. He was also pointing to the climber above him so that the helicopter team would understand that he was the one who needed rescuing.

'Want me to drop you on the summit?' asked Gérard.

'No. By the time we set up the winch he'll already be at the bottom. He's only holding on with his axes and it doesn't look like he could be bothered to put an ice screw in. Can't see why. Best to winch me down to him. I'll attach the sling to his harness, you bring me up again and drop us down on the Col du Midi. Think it'll work?'

'It'll have to!'

The safety rating on the Alouette's winch means it's not supposed to take two people at the same time. Even though it's strong enough to hold two, an essential safety margin makes it inappropriate for that kind of operation. Tony finished putting his crampons on, just in case. In theory, he wasn't going to have to set foot on the ice at all. The only worry was the downwash from the rotor blades. As long as it didn't disturb the little group of people below us too much.

'Ready, Tony?' asked Xav, who was in charge of the winch.

'Yep, I've got to unplug this.'

Tony unplugged his headset from the cabin system and plugged it into his walkie-talkie. This would allow him to talk to Xav with the mouthpiece. In this kind of winching operation, it's in the rescuer's interests to stay in contact with the winch operator at all times, as they only have a few centimetres to play with. Xav's view of what was going on beneath us was foreshortened and he had to be guided by Tony suspended on the hook below.

'Ok. Go. Five metres … ten metres … twenty metres. All right, granddad, stop there. Wait! He looks like he's about to go … No, it's ok. He's hanging on.'

I tried to see what was going on but I was on the wrong side of the chopper. I didn't dare move for fear of upsetting the balance of the machine. I was surprised they hadn't already dropped me off at the Col du Midi to get rid of the extra weight. But there hadn't even been time for that.

Tony was almost at the same height as the solo climber.

'Come in closer to the wall … Three metres …'

Xav was giving Gérard a running commentary on what he could see so that the pilot knew exactly where he was. Gérard in turn was concentrating on the edge of the cornice to hold the helicopter stationary. His mechanic was his eyes. He manoeuvred the joystick with his fingertips, moving metre by metre, trying to anticipate where the gusts of wind would come from. Whatever happened, he simply had to keep the helicopter stationary.

Tony was very close to the solo climber now. Pushing on the radio's button attached to his throat he spoke into the microphone.

'Two more metres … Another metre … Gently! Gently does it, Xav.'

His voice was slightly staccato and he sounded nervous.

Bernie looked petrified. Surprised by the arrival of a rescue that he wasn't expecting, he hadn't put in an ice screw to set up a possible belay. The only thing he had had time to do was place his left axe in the ice and clip himself to it. Braced against the left-hand axe, he had taken the leash of his other axe off and was reaching out to Tony. But Tony didn't want his hand. His main objective was to get as close as possible to the climber, steady himself with his front points in the ice and clip the sling to the central loop on the victim's harness.

'Too far left, Xav, I'll come in right on top of him! Right, Xav, right ... a metre right!'

Bernie didn't understand what was going on. That's the main problem with rescues: the rescuer has to resort to quite a bit of ingenuity to make the victim understand how he is going to help. And all that with the maddening din and wind of the helicopter above.

'That's it, I'm there ... Don't move, Xav,' Tony yelled.

It should all have worked out perfectly to plan, if it hadn't been for one small hiccup. An instinctive reaction, nerves and sheer bad luck sent it all crashing down. Bernie clumsily reached out and tried to grab Tony's arm but as he did so he knocked into the lone ice axe from which he had unclipped himself. The axe tore out of its poor placement and, without thinking, he instinctively tried to catch it with his free hand. At the same time he pushed away from the wall of ice on his good leg. As he leaned out, the angle the sling made with the other axe, and from which he was hanging, opened up. It all happened very quickly.

He swivelled round on his left foot and fell on to his side. The second axe ripped. Seeing the climber go, Tony grabbed hold of his arm but all he felt in his hands was sleeve. He held on to him as best he could, despite the precariousness of his grasp. Suddenly, the cable jolted him to the right. The violence of the tug made him let go of his prey. The climber, to his horror, who had neither foothold nor handhold, felt himself falling backwards. Tony, terror-stricken, watched powerlessly as he fell. He cried out in desperation.

'Shit! Shit! I let go! I let go of him! Fucking hell!'

The rest of us sitting in the helicopter were dumbfounded. We'd never lost anyone like that before.

Tony wriggled around on the end of the cable trying to see where the body would land. He had time to see the two other climbers below. No, this can't be happening. He was going to take out the other two as well. It was horrific.

'Fuck, Catherine, look out. Here he comes!' roared Rémi who just had time to flatten himself against the wall of ice as he saw the lump come hurtling towards him. They were finished. Both of them were going with him. It was all over. Just like in the books, his whole life flashed before him: his kids, university, his wife, plans for the future ... His whole life reduced to a few tenths of a second.

The initial blow was violent. Rémi felt his jacket tear as if it was made of rags. They had a fraction of a second before both of them were going to be catapulted into the abyss. Catherine was crushed under the weight of her companion. Paradoxically, a feeling of powerlessness and fragility had wiped away any anxiety, as if fate had already taken control of the final moments of her life and, in a final gesture of compassion, had taken away all sensation from her.

Then came the second blow. The other climber had literally bounced off Rémi but his boot was caught in a loop of rope that was hanging ten metres below the stance. It should have ripped at that point. But the rope went tight for a moment and then, like an elastic band, it relaxed. Rémi, who had his eyes glued to the two ice screws he had placed, watched as the left one ripped out taking the entire lump of ice it was fastened to with it. That was the one he was clipped to. As one with the block of ice, he fell and found himself hanging from the end of the sling with which he had clipped himself to the ice screw, a metre below. Thank God he had had time to attach a sling from one screw to the next! The other climber wasn't quite so fortunate, and his foot had somehow worked itself free from the loop of rope. His body fell, like a puppet, all the way down the slope, tumbling over and over to the accompaniment of the sound of metal scraping on rock and ice.

A few seconds later he disappeared between two séracs.

Rémi could hear himself breathing hard. His whole body was trembling. Catherine was sobbing. They were both alive, hanging from a single pathetic ice screw in the middle of a mountain face. Rémi stared flatly at the ice screw, at the ice screw that had held them. He thought of the two kids they had almost left orphans. So, there is a God somewhere. But not apparently for the other guy …

'Take me right down to the bottom, I want to see where he is!'

Tony was screaming into his radio. We'd never heard him like this before.

Gérard headed off in the direction of the yawning holes of the séracs whose mouths opened up ravenously towards the Torino hut, on the other side of the massif. Tony followed, flying through the air, still attached to his cable.

There was no way the guy could have possibly survived as he careered down the seemingly endless 65-degree slope, plunging down towards a hanging glacier. The Alouette came to a stop and hovered above the first dark crack. Being slowly lowered down, Tony was scrutinizing the cone of debris at the bottom of the slope, where he was sure to have ended up.

'Lima, lower me down a bit more, I can see him! Further right!'

There he was. He had landed on a plug in the bottom of the crevasse. He was hugging his knees and trying to recover his wits.

'He's alive! Set me down and send Manu.'

'Calm down, calm down! What's your name?' Tony asked the guy who was clearly delirious.

'Yeah, follow me … Take in … Slack, I need slack …'

The guy had no idea who he was or where he was. He tried to get up, then sit down, and then he wanted to turn around. His helmet had flown off his head and landed two metres below him, half his trousers were ripped to shreds and he was vainly battling to try and take off his backpack whose strap was tangled around his shoulder.

'Slowly does it. We're here to help you. What's your name?' Tony asked again.

'Er …'

'Oi! What's your name?' It was my turn to ask.

'Bernie, my name's Bernie!'

'Where does it hurt, Bernie?'

'Go on, more, go on. Take in the rope …'

'Calm down, Bernie. I'm a doctor. Let me do my job.'

Bernie was completely wired but we couldn't afford to hang around here, under this ice chute. We could be hit by lumps of ice or a slide of snow at any moment. We just had to move a little bit, so we weren't right under it. Bernie wasn't having any of it. His face was covered in blood but apart from that he didn't appear to have any major lesions. It was a miracle he was still alive and wasn't, or so it seemed, more badly injured. My main worry, all the same, was for his head. He was exhibiting all the signs of someone who'd had a pretty major crack on the head. The kind of agitation he was showing could also be the sign of internal bleeding. We had to be careful as, given how far he had fallen, we could expect to find just about anything.

'Manu, you've got to give him something,' declared Tony, 'we can't do anything with him like this.'

That was easy for him to say! It would still take a few minutes to give him the injection and wait for him to do as he was told. For the time being he was far from in agreement with us. Every time I tried to roll up his sleeve to find a vein he held out his arm with his hand in a fist and smacked his other hand on to it just above the elbow, swinging his hand up into a time-honoured 'up yours' *bras d'honneur*!

'Tony, call for help. We're never going to manage on our own,' I ordered.

Tony was gesticulating behind Bernie's back and, it wasn't difficult to translate, he meant let's get hold of him, tie him to the stretcher and get out of here. This was the old, quick and dirty method. But this guy was big! My patience finally paid off and I was able to reason with him. He was a little bit calmer now. His sleeve was pushed up and made an impromptu tourniquet. I could see a lovely-looking vein throbbing in the fold of his elbow. I couldn't afford to miss. I carried on talking to him all the time as I approached with the needle of a green catheter.

Each colour of catheter corresponds to a different diameter. The blue ones, for instance, are for children. The orange and grey ones are the large calibre catheters that we use for people in shock, when we need to get fluids into patients as quickly as possible. The green one is the intermediate size. Once the vein has been pierced, the needle is removed leaving the tiny plastic sheath that covers it in place. This tiny tube gives us permanent access to the vein without having to leave the metal needle in, as we used to. In a rescue setting, this avoids having to carry a drip around with us that's sure to freeze or get ripped out as we move around. A special little cap screws on to the tube that sticks up out of the surface of the skin. We can then inject drugs through the tube at any moment.

'Let me do this, Bernie, it's going to hurt a little bit. Ok?'

Success: the needle was in place. I could tell by a backflow of blood in the cannula, it was almost ok. For pity's sake, please stop moving.

'Stop, stop! You bastard, that hurts! Let go of me,' screamed Bernie.

Tony tried to hold his arm as best he could. Bernie wriggled. It was too late. The catheter popped out. Bernie had ripped everything out.

'Shit. For Christ's sake, Bernie!'

Lima was lowering Arnaud down to us. Arnaud's a big bloke and had brought the stretcher with him. I was starting to think Bernie was an ideal candidate for Ketamine. I discreetly set about preparing the syringe, trying not to look like I was preparing a syringe, and attached an intramuscular needle. I briefly summarized the situation to Arnaud who had just arrived.

'Give us a hand. I'm going to inject this in his arse. We've got no choice, I don't fancy hanging around here.'

All the subtlety of anaesthetics rests with giving the patient enough so that they leave us alone but not so much that they stop breathing. I really didn't fancy the thought of getting out all the hardware – intubation kit, respirator and all the rest – this really wasn't the place for all that. The guy probably had slight concussion, a small intracranial haematoma or a few bruises of the grey matter. The kind of thing that can be treated. Fifty milligrams should be enough to be getting on with, it works pretty fast. If the worst came to the worst I could give him a bit more. We still had a little bit of time left, and I could have been criticized for using a drug that was contraindicated for head injury victims. But medicine is a bit like the tides, they come in and then they ebb away again. One day you can get into trouble for using a drug considered toxic for a particular kind of illness, and the next minute you're about to be struck off for *not* using it! It's fashion. That's what's happened with Ketamine. After it was dropped in favour of more modern drugs, it has been rehabilitated and is now an indispensable alternative. A drug that was considered harmful not so long ago is now not so harmful after all. Medicine is the art of not swimming against the tide.

In any case, with Bernie I had no choice. The needle passed through the fabric of his trousers and came to rest in where I estimated his left gluteus maximus was. The efficacious nature of the product was quick to reveal itself. When you need a radical solution, you can't beat it. Bernie had already stopped moving. He became completely stiff, his eyes staring glassily as if he had temporarily absented himself from his thoughts. Ketamine is the drug of virtual sleep; you sleep with your eyes open.

I checked the oxygen saturation of his blood with my little sensor gizmo on the end of his finger: 78 per cent, not bad for an altitude of 3,500 metres but very low for someone with a brain injury. I would have to put him on oxygen as soon as we got into the helicopter. We tied our man up and were all winched into the helicopter. I wasn't sorry to be finally saying goodbye to the place.

Two hours later we were back at the hospital with another patient who had managed to impale himself, ramming a karabiner through his hand as he tried to catch hold of a quickdraw. We found Bernie completely awake and perfectly lucid. He looked at me as if he had never seen me before in his life. I explained that we had already met, probably in another dimension. He must have thought I was a nutter.

His scans were on the x-ray viewer. We could make out a small opaque area under the dome of his skull, nothing particularly serious, a small extradural haematoma that shouldn't get any worse. Another miraculous escape.

I returned home exhausted that evening. My children, Alix and Pierrot, were so excited and worked up that Cécile, my wife, had given up any attempt to try and get them under control. *Plus ça change*! I wasn't faring any better at calming them down. After half an hour of trying to get them to go to bed, I finally managed to kiss them goodnight and turn off the lights.

At the same moment, not far from Grenoble, Catherine was also hugging her children, harder than she had ever hugged them before. She had come close to never seeing them again that day. Life does indeed hang by a slender thread sometimes.

A DIFFERENT KIND OF RESCUE

• • • • • • • • •

It was Wednesday, and I wasn't on call. My daughter Alix and I caught the early train to Paris that morning. At last we were going to collect Khando. It was to be the happy ending to a long and tortuous story.

My wife and I first met Khando a few years before when I was working as a doctor with a film crew in the Dolpo region of Nepal. The little girl was in a bad way, suffering from digestive tuberculosis, undernourished, riddled with parasites. We treated her as best we could before seeing she got to hospital in Kathmandu and, once she had pulled through, we sent money for her food and schooling in the Nepalese capital. I had seen Khando several times since then while on various trips to Nepal. She was now in good health but an orphan so we embarked on the official process to bring her to be educated in France. Adoption didn't seem the ideal solution, but at the same time I felt like the father she had never known. We wanted to see how she adapted to life so far away from home, as we wanted her to live with us during the school year. The understanding was she could return to Kathmandu for the holidays.

The paperwork involved to achieve this was endlessly complicated, not helped by the Nepalese authorities trying to extract backhanders and our helpers in Kathmandu being unwilling to give in to blackmail. I had gone once to Roissy Charles de Gaulle to meet a Royal Nepal Airlines flight, only to find Khando had not been allowed to board. But now, on our third attempt, we had suddenly succeeded and a painter friend called Norbu had managed to bring her to Paris at the last minute.

There she was staying with someone we had only spoken to on the phone called Marie-Jeanne who was deeply involved in the integration of Nepalese people into French society. Our only worry now was that Marie-Jeanne had taken a real shine to Khando and, on two days' acquaintance, seemed to be thinking of adopting the little girl herself. She was certainly loath to let her go and had kept on about Khando needing to feel in her own prayer environment. 'That means she's got a thangka on the wall,' Cécile explained wryly after taking one of her phone calls. Marie-Jeanne sounded completely bonkers to us, and this was why Alix and I were hot-footing it to Paris to collect Khando, whatever it took.

We climbed the stairs of a small suburban apartment block. Alix was anxious to meet her new friend who she only knew from a few photos and my description. Her excitement was turning to anxiety the closer we got and she was getting a stomach ache.

Khando was by the door when it opened. She gave us a mischievous look, her round features leaving no doubt as to her Tibetan ancestry. She was the picture of health and happiness. A far cry from the little Dolpo girl we had treated five years earlier. I couldn't believe my eyes, Khando was finally actually here.

Alix and I gave her a hug and tried out our extremely limited Nepali: '*Tapaailaai kasto chaa?* (How are you?)' She shook her head from side to side and replied '*Sanchai chha!* (Fine!)'

in the disconcerting way the Dolpo have of agreeing with you while seeming to say no.

We greeted Norbu. I was happy to see him again. There were some tense exchanges with Marie-Jeanne and a forced friendliness to the conversation. I was dreading her coming up with a last-minute strategy to stop me from taking Khando away. We weren't going to fight over her. Thankfully, Norbu glossed over all that by explaining to Khando that she would be going to stay with us. Marie-Jeanne, who claimed to speak fluent Nepalese, didn't get a word of it, although she assured us she had. Time was ticking by, but not fast enough for my liking. Alix and I finally managed to tear Khando from the clutches of her jailer, who was seething. I was the one who was going to end up feeling guilty. There were tears and we said a final few goodbyes as we hastily turned to walk away before she came after us.

Khando and Alix played together in the train and they were already friends. It was ok, she didn't seem to miss Marie-Jeanne. The TGV sped on to Bellegarde. The girls had started on an impressive drawing session, giggling as they swapped pictures. They had very different styles.

Comforted by the rocking of the train as it raced through the night, I recalled the things that had happened to me on the other side of the planet. I thought about the rescues in which I had been involved. My work is normally regulated by a series of short adventures, fleeting episodes in the chronicles of mountaineering, a bit like video clips. Like the climber who in the prime of life takes a fall and cracks his skull open. I come down out of the sky clipped to my steel cable, the guy doesn't see me and I don't know him. I harness him up to my more or less miracle-working tubes and whisk him off as quickly as possible to some anonymous hospital facility. I leave again as soon as I can, trying to remember all my equipment.

I never see the majority of accident victims ever again. They are either dead or they don't want to relive the nightmare by seeing me again. Sometimes, it is a sense of reserve, a feeling of guilt at having made a nuisance of themselves, that holds them back. Or it is embarrassment at the thought of been laid bare while unconscious. Other times they can't remember a thing or they don't care.

I like it when one story stands out from the everyday, from the brief encounters of rescues. When there is a sense of continuity with echoes through time and consequences. A life saved then regains its value.

Khando's story is one of these essential experiences. There aren't many in a rescuer's career but thanks to them all the other rescues, about which you never hear another word, take on the happy ending you wish you had known.

I had to journey deep into the Dolpo region to realize that, far from my usual microcosm, being a doctor is no longer just a question of professional status. It's a permanent and universal state of being. It sticks to you and you can't separate it from your identity, wherever you are and for whatever reason you find yourself there. Such as in the path of a malnourished girl somewhere in the heart of the Himalaya.

We took on the little Dolpo girl out of compassion or perhaps duty, without knowing or considering what would happen next. Cécile is true to herself and her word, and adopted Khando in three words and three movements. It took no more than a week for Khando to become part of our family.

BIG CHIEF

• • • • • • • • •

We live in the Ecole de Taconnaz. It's an old school that we did up with our own sweat and tears. Cécile requisitioned the whole of the first floor to do bed and breakfast. When we bought it a dozen or so years ago, all that was left inside was the old blackboard, which we kept hold of so that the kids could scribble on it instead of the walls.

It was the beginning of March, the busiest month for ski tourers, freeride enthusiasts skiing the steepest slopes in the massif and mountaineers on snow routes.

Seven-forty-five. The phone rang. Although above-average temperatures were forecast, it was still pretty cold in the house. The phone was obviously on the wrong side of the bed as it woke Cécile up first. With all our obligations and nights on call for her the nurse and me the doctor – I know, we make a pretty conventional couple – we had lost track of who was supposed to be on duty.

As it happened, it was for me. Benzalès's booming voice woke me from a weird dream where I was fighting off a cloud of flies.

'Manu? It's Marcel.'

'Um, yeah …'

It was too early in the morning for a smart riposte.

'We've got a recce to do. Looks like a team might have fallen off the Swiss Route on the Courtes, above the bergschrund.'

He might be wide-awake but I wasn't.

'Yeah … Right … I'm on my way.'

Still half asleep, Cécile managed a few words of encouragement.

'What is it?'

'Bugger. What is it with these people? Why do they have to fall off things so early in the morning?'

On the landing before heading downstairs I could hear snoring coming from the girls' room. Whether she was in her native Dolpo or here in Taconnaz, Khando had a perpetually runny nose.

And we were off again. I had a spluttering radio in the pocket of my not-so-yellow Patagonia jacket, my pack in the boot, morphine in my bum bag and a CD of *Dancing in the Dark* playing to wake me up gently.

As usual, the pilot had been scrambled first, then the rescue team and at the last moment someone had said, 'Hang on, where's the doc?' Hence I arrived in a complete rush as everyone else was already in the chopper. To let me know how late I was, the rotor blades on the Sécurité Civile's Alouette helicopter were already spinning. I barely had time to pull my harness on before throwing myself into the helicopter. All that so as not to get a bollocking!

'Hi, Dragon,' I said the second I had my helmet on.

But they didn't have time to reply: we had had a call from the Argentière hut.

'Hi, Joseph, we're listening.'

Joseph, the hut's guardian, had some pretty funny ideas about rescues but he was a good shepherd to his flock of mountaineers. Among other things, he was also quick and to the point when it came to filling us in on an accident.

'Right, there's three of them. One's moving and the other two aren't.'

Brief though it was, his description told me a great deal about the work expected of me.

We arrived at the bottom of the Swiss Route and the Alouette delicately set a skid down on one of the mounds of snow left by the sluff that must have accompanied the climbers on their long glissade.

'Right, out you jump.'

We jumped down one after another, like parachutists but from a smaller height. The gear followed, with not such a soft landing. We sank up to our knees in lumpy snow. The avalanche had gone surprisingly early in the morning but it was supposed to be unseasonably warm that day and the Swiss Route gets the sun early.

The survivor who was able to move looked a bit shocked, which was hardly surprising, given the fall he had just taken. He looked haggard, as if he had just been hit by lightning. His face was swollen, he had a black eye and his hair was decidedly dishevelled. He still had snow on his head and, as is often the case, the lower parts of his trousers had been ripped to shreds by his crampons.

'Are you French?'

'Yeah, I'm from Argentière!'

'Are you in any pain?'

'Er... I don't really know...'

He said something else but the helicopter was right above us and I couldn't hear a word. As he didn't seem to be a big problem, we put him in the helicopter to save it going back down empty.

The others were a whole different ball game. There's nothing more complicated than making a rapid assessment of two patients at once, especially when they're tangled up in their rope, half-strangled by slings and rucksack straps. They were completely straitjacketed.

All I could say was that they were groaning. So, they were alive. The best thing to do in these situations is calm everyone down. It's not always easy when some rescuers are convinced it's a race against time. It was a nice day and the mountains were looking spectacular and we would be kidding ourselves if we pretended going faster would resolve anything. So I got out my penknife and started cutting away at the bits of rope. It breaks my heart to wreck gear like that. As a climber I know how much it costs.

We were just about getting there, when one of the rescuers shouted, 'Out the way! There's another sluff coming.'

We rushed ten metres to the right to get out of the way of the avalanche that buried one of the victims who, for obvious reasons, couldn't get away with us.

At that moment I realized I had forgotten my ARVA. We really ought to remember to have these avalanche transceivers with us all the time, even in summer.

'Ok, let's get back to work.'

We ran back to dig out the buried victim who was starting to suffocate and was still wrapped up in his ropes. He looked a bit out of it. As always, my role was to make an initial evaluation

of the type and severity of the trauma, and its potential seriousness, to give the victim a shot of something, get an IV-line
going, in order to give fluids and resuscitate him if necessary.

The first of the two patients clearly belonged in the multiple
injuries category: with a broken wrist, one or two broken ver-
tebra and a few fractured ribs, he wasn't too bad. The other guy
was looking a little less cooperative. He kept pushing the
oxygen mask off as the rescuer tried to hold it over his nose.
The man looking after him had tried his best to calm him down,
but there was nothing to be done, the guy was suffering.

I decided not to waste too much time with the first victim. I
opened my bum bag in which I had just enough to make a catheter and give him something for the pain. That way I didn't
have to open my rucksack that I kept for major damage. I
spotted a good-looking vein zigzagging under the skin on the
back of his hand. Just because they look good it doesn't mean
we can't miss them. And I missed this one and a lump immediately came up. Serves me right for being too cocky. I was
irritated now as I was going to have to find another vein higher
up his arm and the sleeve of his jacket was in the way. It always
pains me to have to cut open a 400 euro jacket. I took a good
minute to make sure I properly prepared this vein, patting it
and rubbing it with alcohol. It was much smaller and less
obvious than the first one but this time I was spot on. I stuck it
down with a bit of transparent adhesive and gave him a quick
shot of nalbuphine to keep him quiet until we got to hospital.
It's a derivative of morphine we use on a daily basis which has
the advantage of leaving the injured person more or less
cooperative.

I called Kevin over. He was the young rescue guy with me.

'Can you watch him for two seconds, the time it takes for the drug to kick in? I'll have a look at the other one.'

The second patient wasn't looking very good and I regretted not dealing with him first. Unfortunately it often happens that way: we go to the victim who screams the loudest first, while the other one is quietly croaking in the background.

Sure enough, he was going under. His helmet had come off and he definitely looked like someone who was going to need intubating. That said, with a bit of luck he might pull through. In cases of people sliding for hundreds of metres over hard snow, head injuries are not always due to a single violent impact but can be the result of a series of blows. We call it the milk shake effect. The brain swells up due to repeated shaking. A scanner will show generalized oedema without a localized lesion. If there is not too much swelling the patient will often go on to enjoy a complication-free recovery.

Intubation in the field is something you can never perfectly master and anyone who say otherwise is a liar. While it's rare for it to go wrong in the sterile environment of the operating room – where there's good lighting, alternatives in case it goes wrong, and the patient has an empty stomach – the delicate procedure of intubation is a great deal more tricky in the inhospitable mountain environment. Out there you're on your own and you can't rely on the mountain rescue team to help you get the tube in, as it's not their job. It doesn't happen often enough for them to be comfortable with it. You're lying in snow or on rocks and your equipment has a habit of scattering itself around you. It's often freezing cold and wet. The helicopter is constantly overhead, bringing up gear required in the rescue. It feels like you're in a war-zone. If the patient hasn't eaten, all the better. If they've eaten, there's a real risk of them vomiting breakfast all over your face. In short, intubation is a far from simple procedure and you really have to weigh up the pros and cons of doing it in the mountains. Sometimes the need to speed off to a more appropriate environment will get the better of you. We call this an American-style scoop and run.

I was pleased, as it seemed to have gone to plan this time. I got a good catheter into the fold of his arm and managed to inject him with the usual cocktail of etomidate and celocurine. The first drug is a strong sedative that completely disconnects you from reality. The second is a curare that paralyses all the muscles in your rib cage and opens the glottis just long enough for a laryngoscope to go through. This is known as a crash induction.

A minute later my patient started to tremble, which is a normal reaction to the curare. Then his jaw relaxed.

It's in this instant that a doctor realizes the extent of his power: to have these kinds of drugs at his disposal and, moreover, the right to use them always seems incredible to me. But it's a double-edged sword, as at that moment everything depends on the doctor. The eyes of the entire rescue team are on the medic, which doesn't make the task any easier, especially if he or she is new to the job. Even when you have a few years' experience under your belt, there are still plenty of surprises lying in wait.

I moved his tongue out of the way with the laryngoscope, trying not to break a tooth, slid the blade in as far as the epiglottis, pulled downwards and slipped the intubation tube down his trachea like a knife moving through butter.

The rest was just plumbing: all I had to do was tie the tube to the patient, connect the respirator to the oxygen bottle at one end and the patient's breathing tube at the other. He could stop breathing and the machine would take care of it!

Another emergency call came in as we were taking our patient from the Courtes back down to the valley. There was no way we could fly him to Geneva, that would take the helicopter at least two hours and that didn't include the time it would take to fill up back at the DZ. The fuel reserves are limited. At altitude, the pilots tend only to take enough fuel in the tank for the mission, to keep the machine as light as possible and maximize its capabilities.

The nearest neurosurgical centre to Chamonix for referrals, so to speak, is in Geneva. We are supposed to be affiliated to Lyon and Grenoble but they are too far to fly with the helicopters we use for rescues. To do it properly, we would have to be able to call the neurosurgeon on duty from the accident site and organize the admission of the patient while also organizing the hand-over of the patient to a second helicopter, leaving the first one available for rescues in the massif. But two times out of three we are left hanging on the phone for a quarter of an hour as we wait to speak to the house officer. It takes him or her a further half an hour to find the surgeon, who in turn will not be able to respond immediately. So, after listening to the entire repertoire of music on hold, we finally give in and call the cantonal hospital in Geneva.

Geneva's cantonal hospital is, of course, in Switzerland, hence it is expensive. Nevertheless, in the absence of a specialist centre nearer us in France, the French social security authorities, which reimburse the fees incurred by its citizens, grant dispensations for the most serious emergency cases.

Ironically, the process is a lot quicker in Switzerland and I have rarely seen them refuse a patient. When we make an emergency call, we are speaking to the triage doctor in around thirty seconds and will have a response within fifteen minutes. An hour later the patient is being cared for in Geneva. The other advantage is that we can often take the patient there directly, without having to change helicopters.

Huge amounts of energy are expended at the pre-hospitalization stage to get places for difficult cases in the best equipped specialist centres, which are also the most expensive. To think that our patients are commodities we have to talk up to get them referred. Try telling that to their families!

Today's victim from the Swiss Route would be going to the Chamonix hospital. Not because the second rescue was urgent, we were collecting a couple of exhausted climbers, but because we had to move quickly to collect the two rescuers we had left at the foot of the Courtes. Dragon dropped me off with my patient and went back to the DZ to refuel.

It was the holidays and all the cubicles in the emergency department were full. The place was crawling with people. As ever, as soon as an interesting case pops up, the entire staff – non-residents, trainees, foreign residents and student nurses – turn up and get under each other's feet in the small emergency room.

My patient lay there oblivious to the mayhem around him. The fentanyl, an analgesic one hundred times more potent than morphine, I had administered after intubating him had plunged him into a restful sleep. Nothing further was asked of him and the machine was breathing for him, providing more oxygen than he could want. He was quiet and, at the very least, compliant. He was waiting for us to unload him from the Piguilhem mountain rescue stretcher.

The transfer of the patient in the emergency department is an important moment. It is the first direct contact the victim has with the care team. The latter has members with a range of different abilities: there are those who know what they're doing and those who only think they know. There are those who are in a rush, those who are completely on the ball, those who get stressed about it and those who seem half asleep through it all. Everyone is waiting for somebody else to give the orders to unload the patient. And when the signal is given, without fail, there's always something – a strap, karabiner, the patient's harness or the intubation tube – that gets caught as we're holding the patient above the stretcher.

Once he or she is on the clean sheets of the emergency room trolley, the real show gets underway. The routine is well-rehearsed as everyone knows more or less what they have to do: undress the patient, get a second line in, attach all the tubes, hook him up to a heart monitor, check the blood oxygen saturation levels and blood pressure and so on.

Generally, there will also be a secretary running around, trying to get hold of the patient's contact details. That's progress for you: no contact details, no computer record and no treatment. But we shouldn't complain, we don't yet ask our patients for their credit cards in France. Luckily for him, our patient wasn't Czech or Korean and had the good sense to leave his identity card in his bag.

Now it was time to tell my colleagues all about the patient. But it wasn't my lucky day. The new A&E doctor had only been here a few days. He hadn't bothered to say hello, so

neither did I. Apparently he was from Lyon. I would have preferred one of my mates. At least with them I wouldn't have to
justify myself and waste three hours explaining what I had
done. We do the same job. With this new guy, on the other
hand, it looked like I was going to have to start at square one.

For a start, it didn't look like he knew what a crevasse was
and secondly, he didn't seem to know anything about climbing. Not like the usual team. In fact, he rather fancied himself
as a hotshot skier because he could get down black runs in Val-
Thorens! I decided to be polite, reminding myself I used to be
in his shoes.

But no, he immediately irritated me with his stupid questions.

'You didn't put a nasogastric tube in?'

The question seemed so off-wall that all I could respond
was, 'Er no, what for? I was on a mountain. You can put one in
now, if you like.'

'What drugs did you give him? He looks completely out of
it to me.'

That one got me and I shot back at him, 'Ketamine ... Horse
Ketamine.'

He eyed me suspiciously. I exchanged a knowing glance
with one of the nurses. Apparently, he wasn't very popular. He
must have come from some big city emergency department.
This pedantry was going to get on everyone's nerves, starting
with Big Chief. I could already hear the sound of his long
stork-like legs striding down the corridor. With his hands
clasped behind his back and his gown flapping open, he left
little eddies in his wake.

His footsteps slowed as he approached the resuss room. He
stood a whole head above everyone else. The staff immediately

went quiet. Big Chief really liked it when that happened! He ignored the Lyon doctor and, glancing at the patient, asked with an amused look, 'What have you brought us this time, Emmanuel?' Deliberately emphasizing each syllable like an old schoolmarm. It was his way of putting us at ease.

'Erm, that ...' I said, motioning to the patient with my chin.

'Yes, and where did 'that' fall from?'

'It's the 'Courting' season and there's always a bit of sliding around up there.'

'And did your patient get very far before the fall?'

'I dunno, he didn't say. In any case, he and his mates jumped the bergschrund. Given the time, I guess they were on their way up.'

He glanced at the tube sticking out of my man's mouth and said, 'I see you've finally managed to get them in the right hole now.'

Git!

The bloke from Lyon didn't say a word. He was looking a bit pale. For an instant I almost felt sorry for him. It wasn't his jargon, this wasn't what he was used to and he was out of his depth. He was thrown completely off balance. It was very simple, he didn't exist any more; it was as if he had already been fired.

Big Chief took me to one side and said rather laconically, 'He's all right, the new boy, isn't he? What do you think? He seems to know his doctoring and is very experienced ...'

I looked discreetly over at the pot-belly and short legs of the man from Lyon. I have to admit that I couldn't really see him working at the bottom of a crevasse, no matter how much he worked out.

Turning back to me, Big Chief added out loud and with a slightly mocking tone, 'Right, well, seeing as your colleague is from Lyon and has a great [he seemed to put excessive emphasis on the word 'great'] deal of experience, he'll be able to find our man a spot in a neurosurgical ward, in Lyon, for example!'

I love it when Big Chief does his act like this. A masterpiece. Big Chief with his patrician bearing had given a Royal Command Performance.

With time we have become good friends. Like father like son, my boy is best friends with his son. The pair of them together would beat us hollow at almost any video game. Having said that, computers aren't really my cup of tea.

I have had a few memorable moments in the mountains with Big Chief. He was unquestionably the master in the resuscitation room, but I learned that he too had his weaknesses. These exposed themselves little by little, the higher up we got, and were inversely proportional to the air pressure.

Big Chief suffered very badly from acute mountain sickness. A few years earlier we gave ourselves a bit of a scare on an ascent of the Armand Charlet Couloir on the north face of the Aiguille Verte. We had no real problems on the technical ice section at the start of the climb, except once we had done it and realized there was no way we could descend back down the same way. The route's exit follows a snowy couloir for 500 metres to the summit at around 4,000 metres, before a series of abseils on the other side take you down to the Talèfre glacier.

I sensed Big Chief was less talkative than he had been at the start. I was acting as guide and was leading. He often allowed me both the honour and the responsibility. I started breaking trail up the straight snowy gully, trying my best to stay at a steady pace, not too fast but not too slow. Big Chief was slowing down noticeably. Knowing the pace he set at lower altitudes, I started to worry.

At 3,500 metres Big Chief brought up his first snack. At 3,700 metres he vomited his breakfast. At 3,750 metres it was his dinner from the night before. At 3,780 metres I brewed up some tea so that he had something to puke at 3,785 metres. At 3,800 metres my gas canister was empty and Big Chief didn't have anything left in his stomach. His skin looked like parchment, like someone who was clearly very dehydrated. It took us three hours to get to the summit col and Big Chief was running on empty. It was dark and an icy wind had got up but I had to let him rest before starting down the complicated descent on the other side. We had an endless series of abseils to get down over 400 metres of mixed ground. I huddled in a hole while my boss fell into a deep torpor. I was unable to sleep, I was shivering so much, and I made regular checks as to my companion's health, asking him how he was feeling. I suggested that I go down and get help, so that we could be picked up at first light, but he kept telling me he just wanted to sleep. He was slouched in the snow, apparently oblivious to the drop in temperature and the cold tearing through us.

The following few hours seemed like they would never end. By midnight Big Chief wasn't making a sound and I was really worried. If we waited until morning he was going to be seriously hypothermic. I shook him to get him to stand up, which was no easy task. The descent was torture but at least we were out of the wind and not so cold. Every quarter of an hour I told him it was just altitude sickness and all we had to do was lose height and everything would be fine. He gave me a complete earful each time, whingeing right up until we set foot on the glacier. The altimeter on my watch said 3,500 metres and day was breaking.

He looked at me, his spirits considerably improved and said, 'Hey, I don't feel sick any more!'

Eager to regale each other with similar tales, we repeated the experiment several times. It took us a whole thirty-six hours to climb the north face of the Droites via the Tournier Spur. At precisely 3,500 metres Big Chief presented me with exactly the same scenario: vomiting, asthenia and torpor. We were forced to bivouac in the middle of the mountain, what joy! We still managed to do the route and, as on the previous occasion, he perked up considerably once we were on the other side of the mountain, both feet firmly planted on the Talèfre glacier.

Our most recent adventure to date was quite chilling. We took Michel, the friend with whom I had made such a brilliant attempt on the Matterhorn, to do the Nant Blanc Route on the west face of the Aiguille Verte. We moved together on the first section, which didn't have any particularly tricky climbing. Despite the fact Big Chief was the only one of us to have done the route before, back in the good old days, Michel and I swapped leads. The weather wasn't very good and there was a low cloud base, but the forecast was supposed to be good. At the top of the first third of the route we couldn't agree where the line, which seems so obvious when you look at the face from Chamonix, went. Michel and I wanted to join a gully heading left but Big Chief insisted we carry on straight up. A great discussion ensued, but he had done the route before, his voice carried further than ours and he was still the 'boss', so we ended up doing as he said. An hour later we found ourselves in a complete nightmare, crossing, as carefully as we could, great slabs of sliding snow to rejoin the route. We all accused each other of incompetence. Big Chief saw fit to shoulder some of the blame himself. To crown it all, a *cousse*, or drizzling mist, which had been engulfing the summit of the Verte since the morning, gently descended down to where we were. We had wasted a good three hours on a small part of a route that we thought we would get done in a day. Good sense dictated that we call a helicopter now, before the weather socked in completely and as we neared the 3,500-metre mark and Big Chief started to get the first symptoms that he and I knew so well.

The helicopter crew sent down Giulio, a specialist in tricky operations, who had us out of there in next to no time. Unluckily for us Crampon-danger-man was on duty that day and he gave us a right earful. And he still talks about it today!

This last adventure and the thought that acute mountain sickness is after him, has put a dampener on Big Chief's climbing ambitions. He has turned his hand to DIY. Memories and contemplation are what sustain him now.

My radio started whining.

'Come in, Crampon-doc, Dragon calling.'

'Yeah, what is it?'

'Are you ready to go? We've got another rescue.'

'What is it?'

'A Czech on the Tacul with a broken leg. We've got Jansé and will pick you up on the way.'

I got out as soon as I could. I was happy not to be on duty at A&E that day, there were too many people. It didn't look much like fun and there was a morbid atmosphere. I took to the skies again in my steel bird.

Crouching on the hospital landing pad, I didn't even watch the helicopter do its one-eighty above my head while making its hellish racket. The huge beast doing a 'touch and go' is a pretty impressive sight, but not a very unusual one for us, the rescuers. Bystanders watch stock still, doors slam and children look on open mouthed. Meanwhile, inside, the helmet and headset goes on, the door closes and, after a final check of the tail, the pilot is already taking off again.

The small hospital on the edge of the mountains shrank beneath the helicopter. I watched, deep in thought. Its unusual shape made me think of the hammer and sickle of the flag of the Soviet Union. Was that a coincidence? The hospital had spent twenty years resisting repeated assaults from conquistadors in the plain. It had had to fight for its independence and had always had a revolutionary side. A core of hardliners, who were a little arrogant, criticized and revered in equal measure.

BLADES IN THE SNOW

• • • • • • • • •

'According to the guide who called, it happened at about 3,800 metres, level with one of the first séracs. But the weather's pretty iffy. I don't think I can put you down there,' the pilot, Michael, informed us.

Cordial continued the story, giving us more details over the radio from HQ.

'Come in, Dragon, this is Cordial.'

'Yeah, we're listening.'

'Have you left the hospital?'

'Affirmative. Do you know any more about the injuries?' asked Michael.

'Well, a guy jumped the bergschrund and has got a displaced fracture of the leg.'

'Do we know where they are?'

'Yep, one of the guys from the group went down to the Cosmiques hut to sound the alarm. Marianne spotted them with the binoculars. They're at the top, below the shoulder, at about 3,800 metres.'

The Aiguille du Midi disappeared under our feet, its balconies full of tourists. There was quite a bit of turbulence. The weather obviously wasn't going to help. It looked like it might be a bit tricky on the Tacul, there were big and very mobile cumulus clouds converging on the summit. There were strong winds. Michael had a hacking cough. He had abruptly dropped the Senegalese accent he liked to put on when everything was going well. It was a souvenir from equatorial Africa where he had done his basic training.

'I don't know how we're going to do this. We'll try coming from below first.'

Michael wandered all over the place, diving down and climbing back up the slope, zigzagging and slaloming, but it didn't work. He tried from above, but it was the same deal, it was impossible to set us down on the shoulder. He finally suggested dumping us as high as possible up the slope.

On our first approach we were at about 3,300 metres. The clouds came in rapidly and we were brutally enveloped. Jansé jumped out of the machine without any hesitation. Michael had lost his bearings and pulled back away from the ground as soon as possible. He came in for a second attempt to try and drop me off this time. The clouds had come in again and everything was white. There was a 30-degree slope and one of the blades brushed the snow. I jumped into the squall, managing not to swear as I did. I found myself up to my thighs in snow, crushed under the weight of my rucksack. I flattened myself, under the impression I had narrowly missed decapitation. The great beast flew off, leaving me alone in a heavy silence of foreboding. It was snowing. Jansé, who was forty metres above, shouted to me, 'Hey, did you see the blade marks?'

I climbed up towards him, wading through powder snow. Then I saw the horizontal slice in the fresh snow, made by the rotor blades of the Alouette. I swallowed, terrified. The job can be pretty bloody dangerous sometimes!

Here were the two of us, abandoned on the face with a stretcher weighing twelve kilos and our packs full of gear. The injured climber was at least 600 metres higher up and the weather was completely socked in. Jansé called Cordial to explain the problem. A helicopter evacuation or a rescue party on foot? They were going to have to sort something out down there and give us a hand.

'So, what do we do?' I asked

'Start climbing?'

'Yeah, but what are we going to do with the stretcher?'

I didn't see us dragging the whole thing up over 600 metres on a slope loaded with fresh snow, carrying our twelve-kilo packs.

'We'll have to leave it. The others can pick it up on the way. We'll start putting a track in. That's going to be hard enough,' said Jansé.

I followed him up the slope, more or less in agreement.

Jansé was one of the next generation. He was a guide and was newly promoted. He was a bit of a dreamer, with blond hair and blue eyes. He didn't really fit the classic image of a gendarme-rescuer from the seventies. He climbed 8a but that didn't stop him being discreet about it. To think I'd been trying for the past twenty years to climb harder than grade 7 and he was fifteen years younger than me. His girlfriend was pretty and friendly. The pair of them looked like they had stepped out of a chewing gum ad, especially when you saw them in the Berlingo they had converted into a camping car. When I was twenty I too always had something to eat, a sleeping bag and, more importantly, my climbing gear in my Talbot van. I felt old sometimes.

Jansé's girlfriend was a junior officer in the gendarmerie. She and another gendarme would sometimes turn up at A&E because of a road accident or a mugging. As we knew each other we would kiss each other on the cheek when we met (as we do here in France). I've never had anything against law enforcement officers, it's a job just like any other, but she's the only one I kiss …

I was sweating as I had been walking uphill for an hour. Jansé was still marching along in front, like some kind of husky. From time to time we shouted to try and find our Czechs, but had no response. I let Jansé take the initiative. I try as much as I can to stick to my job as doctor and let the rescuers do theirs. I couldn't say if I knew the north face of the Tacul better than Jansé, given my age, and I didn't care. I was happy to let him get on with it. There's nothing worse than having some old sod on your back telling you what to do.

Finally we heard a shout and could make out a shadow coming towards us. One of the Czech climbers was coming to meet us. We tried to explain things to one another in English. The injured climber was above. Were we supposed to follow him? We weren't sure. We followed him through a menacing labyrinth of unstable séracs. The route crossed snowbridge after snowbridge and although it wasn't insurmountable I couldn't see myself carrying some bloke back down that way. It was still snowing.

'Hello, I'm the doctor.'

The guy was leaning against his pack and looked at me as if I was speaking Chinese. I was going to have to work out for myself what the matter was. Yet it wasn't too difficult to diagnose after seeing his right leg: a semblance of a splint had been cobbled together around his broken ankle that was bent outwards. I removed the splint made from bits of Karrimat. His leather boot gaped open miserably. I unwrapped my gear – tourniquet, alcohol swab, green catheter and cap – and explained that I was going to have to put the ankle back straight to reduce tissue damage and ischemia. I may as well have been talking to a brick wall, he didn't understand a word I was saying, despite nodding in agreement. I also explained how I was going to administer a pain killer, also to reduce the effects of the fracture, through a hollow pointed instrument known as a catheter that would hurt a bit as I would have to stick it in a vein in his arm to inject the morphine. Why complicate things? He was agreeing with me.

I shut up in the end and injected him with some nalbuphine. I waited a couple of minutes before taking hold of the ankle and pulling. There was a crack. It was the classic sound of a bone going back into alignment. It's a sound patients don't like to hear but which delights doctors. The Czech winced but hardly moved at all. They're a tough bunch, the Czechs. Jansé and I fitted a vacuum splint to him.

One might have said that we had done the hard bit, but we still had to get him down to the valley and that was going to be another story.

Jansé called Cordial again for news of a back up team, as it was seven in the evening and time was marching on.

'The Aiguille du Midi cable car has stopped running. Too much wind on top. And the helicopter can't fly as it's totally socked in,' Jansé relayed to me.

'Now we're in the shit! If the eight other guys are stuck down there with the sled, after we've been slogging our guts out up here, we're going to end up getting pretty cold!'

'Yeah, it looks like …'

'Jansé, what if we start taking him down the old-fashioned way? I don't fancy digging a hole for the night, not with the weather they've forecast for the weekend.'

'We've at least got to get him as close as we can to the Cosmiques hut. If it snows all night the face'll be completely loaded.'

This was going to be a DIY rescue. We made do with what we had: Karrimat, ropes, packs and slings. Initially, we had to take him through the séracs. Jansé carried him on his back for a bit and then we improvised a kind of rope tow. We struggled, exhausted, like this for over an hour and a half. The guy's mates could have helped but given the amount of gear they had to carry, what with their own and his, we quickly realized that it wasn't going to be possible. We had to manage on our own.

Once past the sérac band, it didn't look like it would be very easy to use the same technique to take the injured climber down the slope that was starting to seriously fill with snow. We were scared it was going to avalanche on us. Plus, it was inconceivable we were going to be able to get through the powder snow with eighty kilos on our backs. We requisitioned all available Karrimats, of which, luckily for us, the Czechs had an impressive stock. We also got out the patient's sleeping bag and wrapped him up in it. Finally, we pulled his hat on his head and fashioned handles at either end of our 'sausage'. Jansé set up a really dynamic belay, as we didn't think the deep snow would hold a huge fall. And I set off with our Czech, attached to the upper sling to push or pull him depending on the terrain.

It didn't go too badly to start with. Our team was shaped rather like a snowplough, but we were making progress. The one fault in our system was that our makeshift sled was engulfed in snow. Nevertheless, our Czech was a stoic chap and kept his mouth shut. We'd given him some ski goggles, to look more the part, and his sleeping bag done up under his nose kept the damage to a minimum. According to the latest from Cordial, the wind had dropped around the Aiguille du Midi and the second team was waiting for the cable car being specially put on for the rescue. At the rate we were progressing, we were going to get to the bottom of the Tacul before them.

But the situation worsened more quickly than we had anticipated. The night fell around us like a lead cloak and my radio gave up the ghost, having run out of batteries. Then the problems started. I knew that the Tacul isn't nice around its lower third. Two almost vertical slopes disappear into two deep bergschrunds, which aren't particularly wide but are big enough to gobble up a doctor and his patient. The problem was I didn't know exactly where they were or what condition they were in, as the helicopter had dropped us off above them.

My field of vision had shrunk. I could barely see the snowflakes swirling in the beam of light from my failing headtorch. The slope steepened and the snow became harder and more slippery. Instead of pushing the sled, I found myself pulled along by it. I was sure we were sliding inexorably towards one or other of the bergschrunds. I had to stop the sled to be able to evaluate the situation. Jansé would have to come down to meet me so that we could concentrate on crossing this section.

But Jansé couldn't hear me.

'Jansé, take. Stop paying out the rope!'

No reaction, I felt very alone.

'Jansé, tight rope!'

I continued sliding towards what looked to me like a black chasm. The sled was dragging me along and seemed to be getting heavier and heavier. Jansé couldn't hear me because of the blasts of wind. Or maybe he was daydreaming, thinking he was rock climbing in a T-shirt in the Verdon Gorge with his girlfriend.

Meanwhile I was shouting myself hoarse.

'Block, Jansé, blooooooock!'

Still no reaction. I only had two solutions left: either continue sliding towards the bergschrund in the hope that in exactly the spot where I was headed it was filled in, or brace myself until I couldn't take it any more. But if I let go at any moment, I would hit any snowbridge that might be there with such force that we were bound to fall through. My patient and I being swallowed up by the bergschrund was hardly an enchanting prospect. Neither was the thought of transforming our support party into a crevasse rescue team. Faced with this perspective, the old survival reflexes took over: I furiously sank my ice axe into white ice with my left hand and cut two paltry steps for my crampons and held the sled with my right hand.

The poor Czech in the sled looked bewildered. As his hands were tied up inside his sarcophagus he couldn't help but he still wasn't complaining. He doubtless had no idea he was suspended above a deep bergschrund with only me holding on to him. As we were attached to each other, we were in this together. We faced the same fate, being squashed to a pulp at the bottom of the bergschrund.

The force of hanging on was going to dislocate my shoulder and I was still yelling, hoping Jansé would snap out of his lethargy. He must have been wondering why the rope wasn't tight any more. I couldn't even radio him as I had both my hands full. In any case, the battery was dead. Suspended and running out of strength, I wasn't expecting anything in particular apart from the moment when I let go. The violent shockloading of two eighty-kilo bodies falling would rip out the belay, and Jansé with it. Then everyone would be in the crevasse.

You should never give up hope, as there is always an answer. I was waiting for the light and it came. Not at the end of the tunnel, but from below the bergschrund. A shaft of light appeared. It wasn't Jansé who answered my cries but another voice, which I recognized and which was coming up from below.

'Manu, is that you?' said the little light.

'Yeah. I'm really in the shit … Who's that?'

'Fabrice. We're coming. What's up?'

'Any minute now the stretcher and I are going flying into the bergschrund. Jansé can't hear a thing. I've got no radio left and I'd prefer it if he held me tight rather than giving slack. Can you do something?'

'Jansé, this is Fabrice.'

He had got out his warm radio.

'Yes, Fabrice, I'm listening.'

'Take, Jansé. Manu's suspended over the bergschrund.'

Almost instantaneously, as if by a miracle, the rope connecting us to Jansé became tight. A great, and unexpected, relief.

Fabrice and the other rescuers had reached the foot of the wall. They climbed up left on the slope of white ice through which the normal route passed. With three of us pulling on the sled, we managed to divert it from its catastrophic trajectory. I wasn't upset to be getting off so lightly.

We got back to the Aiguille du Midi in good spirits. Like the seven dwarves coming home in the dark of night, we pulled the sled through the deep snow. There was a lot of it and even with ten of us it was really hard work, but it wasn't dangerous any more. We weren't singing but we were chattering away like a bunch of schoolgirls. The talk was mainly about techniques, gear, rock shoes and the like. A rescuer who had been coughing for the past four days was desperate for my opinion, as he might have caught tuberculosis … Another one told me he was suffering from a pain in his right shoulder, which was stopping him from going to the climbing wall three times a week. I advised him to stop pulling on it so hard.

Times had changed. When I started out fifteen years earlier, the rescuers were gruff and not very talkative tough types. They didn't climb 8b and didn't chat up lots of girls. We were still in the days of old-fashioned rescues: we walked more and thought less. Or in any case, we didn't ask ourselves existential questions. These days they are more high-maintenance. Some of them come in the high-level athlete category. They are highly tuned machines but break more easily. Some of them even have something of *Top Gun* about them. In short, some are better while others are worse.

The Col du Midi feels big when you are dragging a sled. Discussion moved round to more practical matters like how to get the injured climber back down to Chamonix. Giulio hit upon a clever idea: why not set up the Paillardet electric winch on the top of the Aiguille du Midi. We still had 250 metres of vertical height gain to reach the top. Don't think we had got work-shy over the years, equally don't labour under the misapprehension that a multipurpose rescue sled slides through the snow like a bobsleigh, especially not through fresh powder at an altitude of 3,800 metres! I was so exhausted by the time we reached the Poubelles Couloir I was blessing Giulio. It was eleven o'clock at night and we were all in agreement on his winch idea. An hour later we had all been winched up and were in the lift down, absolutely knackered, but happy. Through the steamed up cable car windows we saw Chamonix by night getting closer. My goatee was still frozen and we were dripping with sweat. From the noise in my eardrums, I knew that the oxygen was gently flowing back into my little grey cells. It was only when we got to the bottom that I realized we had forgotten to untie our Czech. He was still bundled up and hadn't said a word. When I asked him if he was ok he replied, '*Dobje, dobje!* (ok, ok!).'

In fact, we quite like rescues on foot, especially when they're over. The rescue had taken ten of us almost nine hours at an altitude of over 3,000 metres. All that for a simple dislocated fractured ankle. It would have taken two of us half an hour to sort it out with a helicopter. That's the irony of mountain rescues. We are used to how easy they can be, right until a good dose of reality steps back into the arena. Without helicopters, mountain rescues are all about heroism. And it will be a few years before technology allows us to dispense with hard work and dedication in the job.

It was almost warm at one o'clock in the morning in the car park below. Everyone was mucking around before heading off, chuckling. An ambulance was there to take the injured climber to A&E. I made a sign meaning goodbye and he smiled back.

'*Dobje?*' I asked.

'*Dobje!*' came the reply.

It must mean 'ok'. Then again, who knows, it might mean 'dickhead'...

I went home exhausted but pleased, as if the fact that I had taken part in a rescue that was more demanding than normal would mean I got a few days off work. I knew very well that it wasn't going to happen, as we prefer to work in blocks of days so that we can have longer periods of time off. So that we can go into the mountains, for instance ...

Dina and Daisy were waiting for me back at the house. Like all cats, they have an unwelcome habit of constantly rubbing up against your legs and meowing. Their plan is to make you fall flat on your face with the pack full of rescue gear, a radio and a pair of skis in your hand. This is to get you to understand that before looking after injured people in the mountains you really ought to think about giving them something to eat. The mistress of the house must have kicked them out pretty early in the evening and their vole hunt had been fruitless. Dina, the braver of the two, followed my every move. I opened the back door in the kitchen and she ran out, thinking I would bound out after all. She was out of luck, I closed the door behind her. Right, I had got rid of her for the moment. It's not a particularly honourable technique, I know, and it doesn't always work.

I took off my Gore-Tex and unplugged the avalanche transceiver, which would have come in very handy if I had been swallowed up by the dreaded bergschrund. I only had to throw the plate of salt pork and lentil salad in the microwave. I was starving. Feeling guilty, I let Dina back in before eating.

JAMIE

• • • • • • • • •

Sunday, we had no definite plans for the day. It is such a rare occurrence and it feels really good sometimes. I was still worn out from the rescue the day before. We made the most of the sunshine and snow to take the midgets tobogganing. Khando loved it. She had been given any clothes that might fit her and an old-fashioned three-metre scarf trailed behind her. The idea of the game was to find the silliest way of sliding down the slope to the campsite next to the house.

Khando had settled in remarkably quickly. She was very organized and was always doing something. Her first words in French were already coming and her English, basic though it was, was helping. Yet with kids, it is all about contact and interaction and talking is really an adult thing.

My ten-year-old son, Pierrot, was fiercely independent and the presence of Khando in the house didn't change his way of life in the slightest.

It was more complicated for Alix. She was extremely proud of being able to introduce Khando to all her classmates, before being troubled by just how well she settled in. Her position at the heart of the family was being threatened.

Khando put her hand up in class every time the teacher asked anything, even if she didn't understand what was going on. This made everyone laugh. She now had her own friends.

I watched their toboggan contest. I thought how difficult it was going to be for her to return to Nepal. It looked like she liked everything here! Had it been a good idea to bring her to France? She already had to go back the following week. We had explained and explained to her but she didn't want to understand. Her home was here now.

Khando monopolized my thoughts the whole winter, just like Jamie had been on my mind the other winter, when misfortune had descended upon the Chamonix valley like a curse. There had been the fire in the tunnel with its thirty-nine victims burnt alive in atrocious circumstances, deadly avalanches, floods and the infamous tragedy of the two Jamies …

Not far from Scotland a few years ago Jamie was completely inebriated, dancing in his own céilidh. He was drunk but happy. He was also having difficulty staying on his feet, and for good reason; he didn't have any legs. I had my little video camera trained on him. He was my star; since his accident I had become the personal press officer to His Highness the reluctant hero.

I had drunk a fair amount of whisky myself and I wasn't all that sure where I was any more. I was having a few problems focusing. I had no difficulty, however, remembering who the incredible guy gesticulating in the kilt and with the Glengarry on his head was. It was already late and the dance floor was starting to clear but he was still going strong. The band carried on. It was past two o'clock in the morning and Jamie wasn't giving up.

You could see his two metal prostheses clanking together in time to the violin. The girl holding him up must have known him for years. She was roaring with laughter, just letting herself go. I should mention at this point that Jamie has no hands either.

It was the best marriage I had ever been to, apart from my own, of course. He looked great did our Jamie, a real lord.

Anna, his fiancée, had sent an invitation to us at the Chamonix A&E department to the Scottish wedding of a survivor and the woman who never stopped loving him.

I caught the plane with Pascale, one of the nurses who had looked after Jamie during his stay in the hospital. I remembered a noisy journey on a suburban train we had boarded from a deserted platform. There had been a lingering odour of beer. Jamie and Anna were waiting for us, proud of our loyalty. I can still see Jamie masterfully driving with the ball that is fitted to steering wheels for the disabled. The roads were tortuous, bordered by dry stone walls behind which aimlessly wandered flocks of indifferent sheep.

Stranded in a storm on the top of one of the most difficult ice faces in the Alps, the north face of the Droites, in 1999, Jamie had seen his best friend go to sleep for the last time a few metres away from him. They had been caught out, trapped by the mountain. It wasn't through ignorance or recklessness, or through lack of fitness or technique and they hadn't gone off-route. No, it was down to the hard law of the mountains, the accumulation of bad luck and a choice of climbing style.

As always, Jamie and Jamie had decided to weigh themselves down a bit. They took a bit more climbing equipment and bivouac gear, just in case. They had decided to climb 'Scottish-style'. And then the bad weather put its oar in, arriving sooner than had been forecast. The hard ice was utterly draining and slowed them down. They had a first bivouac under the ice couloirs and a second on the summit in a storm. They were suffering badly from exhaustion. They should have started on the descent, two rope-lengths away, dropping on to the other face via a series of abseils to join a more reassuring gully that offers a bit of protection. It is easy to say that when you know. But it wasn't obvious to them. Quite the opposite in fact, and they had nothing left to eat and drink. Everything was frozen, including their hands and feet. So they resigned themselves to a third and then a fourth night of bivouacking.

On the fifth day the clouds split apart and a freezing northerly wind whipped into them. It was a deathly wind, as cold as steel, that turned their last hopes of survival to stone. Jamie Fisher couldn't stand the cold as it bit into his bones and he fell into an ever-lasting sleep. Jamie Andrew knew what had happened and waited his turn. Nothing was going to save him from the white-toothed shark circling round him.

Then there came a humming noise getting louder and louder in the icy air and a 'little blue man' dangling in the sky, buffeted by the wind. Suspended underneath the helicopter, the rescuer grabbed hold of a granite pinnacle sticking up on the right of the col. The helicopter pulled in the cable and Jamie was flying through space. It had been a close one.

The first thing Jamie remembered was a cup of hot tea. The PGHM rescuer was Giulio, a guy who spent his time yomping through the massif. Was it chance or fate? It was perfect that he was on duty for this mission impossible.

Next came the evacuation to the hospital. Was it a dream or was it real? In a matter of minutes Jamie found himself in the stuffy atmosphere so feared by those who are alive and kicking.

It has welcomed through its doors numerous candidates for adventure and frustrated heroes. You love it or hate it; it saves lives or takes them away.

For Jamie it was a place of miracles. First warmth, then light; the silent bustle of the medical team. A short respite before the relapse. First he had to suddenly confront the emptiness: Jamie Fisher, his best friend, was gone. He stared uncomprehending at his lifeless hands and feet. Next a fever set in, he was delirious with blood poisoning. He was surrounded by people taking decisions for him. Finally, came the coma.

It was a slow and difficult awakening. Jamie was a quadruple amputee. We had sacrificed his hands and feet to save his life. His world had been turned upside down. He would never go into the mountains again, no one would ever look at him the same way again. He was so strong and fiercely independent. Must he let himself sink into the world of those dependent on others?

'I will be back!' he had told me in his idiosyncratic French. 'I will come back to see you and I will go into the mountains again!'

'Email me to let me know how you're getting on,' I had replied, not convinced and thinking, how will he type? I didn't see him coming back to Chamonix, not with everything that had happened here.

A year later, I took a chance and sent him a message asking how he was doing. I knew I could. Jamie had so much faith in us that any barriers between the two of us had fallen away. To my great surprise his reply was rapid and with no hang-ups. Unlike most of the English-speakers who visit us, Jamie considered it his duty to speak French even though he had not been taught it. This sometimes led to some surprising results, such as: 'My prosthetic legs and I are getting on very well together, I do 16 seconds at the 100 metres.' He was preparing for the Paralympics.

The following winter Jamie decided to learn to snowboard. On learning this, I suggested he come and practise in Chamonix. I invited him and he came.

Geneva airport, Jamie was beaming. Behind the glass I saw him raise his arms above his head in a gesture of victory. But his hands weren't there any more, it was as if he was showing us he could manage without them, that he was in working order all the same.

Jamie came back to Chamonix the following spring. He had vowed he would climb Mont Blanc ... We were only 300 metres from the summit, buffeted by the wind on the final hump. Since losing his hands and feet, Jamie didn't feel the cold any more and dressed lightly. He was going well, like a real guide – slowly and surely – and he had energy in reserve. A friend of mine, Philippe, was on the other end of the rope, with Jamie in the middle.

We passed two climbers coming down from the summit, their eyes bulging, their faces frozen and looking a bit spooked. It was Nathalie, one of the valley's all too rare female guides, with a client. She was surprised to see Jamie so calm.

'It's stripped bare up there. There are gusts that'll knock you off your feet,' they yelled to us.

Jamie was doubtful. I could sense he was reliving his nightmare and the old ghosts were coming back to haunt him. A violent gust of wind smacked him to the floor. The ridge was becoming ever more tapering. There was a risk ... Jamie still didn't know what to do. I tried to help him make up his mind. I would go along with whatever he decided.

'Jamie, it's your choice.'

It was a long and difficult decision. The wind had strengthened and we were bombarded with tiny particles of hail. Two large and ill-defined clouds menacingly encircled us. I couldn't choose for him, I didn't want to influence him.

'Manu, no. It's too dangerous. It's better to go down. We will do it again another time.'

Jamie was resigned to his decision and it wasn't in his nature to go back on a decision. We turned back, with no sense of bitterness. Happiness wasn't in getting to the end of the road: we had failed, but we were happy.

Jamie and Anna are now part of the family. A little while later, Jamie took his revenge, this time on Kilimanjaro with four other disabled mountaineers from his charity. He sent me a photo from the summit, a pure delight. If it was up to me I would give Jamie a guide's badge. He's been through a great deal more than a lot of us. Me for a start.

FROSTBITE AT THE NORTH POLE

· · · · · · · · ·

I spent an hour evaluating things with Jérôme, the department's only male nurse. He took over responsibility for the medical equipment for mountain rescues. I felt sorry for him and told him so. Having done the job before him, I knew how much hassle it was. Doctors on call for mountain rescues are not really ideal homemakers. You have to be constantly on their backs to get them to tidy away and maintain the shared equipment. Jérôme looked at me, a bit irked that I was already chuckling about it. As we were talking at the end of the corridor, Patricia brought the office phone down to me.

'Manu, it's for you. Frostbite at the North Pole.'

We had been for a few years now *the* centre, of sorts, for the treatment of frostbite and every season two or three people came back from expeditions with black fingers or toes.

I took the receiver she was holding towards me and said in a serious voice:

'Yes, hello?'

'Doctor Cauchy?' asked an unknown voice.

'Yes, this is Doctor Cauchy speaking.' A bit too solemn perhaps.

'Doctor Delange, I work for the Groupama insurance company. Is this a bad time?'

'No.'

'Well, I'm calling you because our group is sponsoring a North Pole explorer. It's Mike Horn, do you know him?'

'No.' Sensing his disappointment I added, 'but it doesn't matter, as I imagine you're going to tell me about him.'

'Yes. He's an explorer on a solo attempt to reach the North Pole completely unaided. He was on the sat phone this morning. His fingers are frozen and he wants your opinion.'

'Er, yes. But where can I meet this brave fellow?' I asked, gently teasing him.

'We're going to have a three way call, if that's ok with you.'

'Really?'

Three minutes later the famous Mike Horn was on the line, lost on an iceberg a few hundred kilometres from the North Pole. His voice was distorted by the satellite connection but the line wasn't too bad. Mike described how his hands looked to me and answered my technical questions. He talked a great deal about his worries and how his frostbite injuries had been looking over the past few days. When he removed his bandages he discovered blisters had formed and the wounds smelt bad. The pads of his fingers were starting to go black. He was worried less about the state of his fingers and more about the prospect of having to call a halt to the expedition when he'd done the hardest part. Given what he had told me, however, I could hardly advise him to carry on. For the time being, he had serious frostbite but it could still heal without complications, if he came home. If he continued, it would get increasingly painful and he would risk amputation.

The decision was an agonizing one for Mike but he eventually decided to continue. I gave him advice on how to limit the damage and he put the phone down.

Two days later Doctor Delange called me back to tell me Mike was on his way home. He had been flown to a small Siberian hospital. According to what the Groupama doctor could make out, the local surgeon already wanted to cut his fingers off. Delange asked me to catch the chartered medical flight to bring Mike home.

I had two days off, so said yes. Picking someone up off the pack ice would make a change from the mountains. The following morning I was waiting for my personal jet to take me across Russia. Leather seats, two pilots, my own personal flight attendant, I could get used to this... A young cameraman, who had been following Mike since the start of his adventure, came along too. I fell asleep soothed by the purring of the engines.

We had a forced landing in Moscow to pick up a third pilot, as no one spoke English where we were going, not even in the control tower of Norilsk airport, our destination. The jet took off again, its fuel tanks full. We commenced our journey over thousands of kilometres of tundra raked by the wind and snow, stretching as far as the eye could see.

We set down on an icy landing strip in the middle of a tiny village that had something of the kibbutz about it. There was no doubt, we were in Siberia. I saw three Russians outside in thick fur coats with impressive ushankas on their heads.

The door opened as we were still in shirt sleeves and we were assaulted by the −40°C cold that froze the hairs in your nose and felt like it was squeezing your head in a vice. I imagined Mike making his way through this kind of atmosphere for over a month. While I thought we were going to take a helicopter and pick him up off the ice pack, it turned out it was he who was going to meet us here but a storm over Dikson Airport was stopping him taking off. It could last for days. Great. We were invited to rest at an establishment that fancied itself as the local Hilton. The antiquated, stifling building had ancient kitsch wallpaper and an enormous noisy dial telephone. On the menu were dry biscuits and boiling coffee juice. We were provided with bedrooms to sleep in but, given the time difference and light streaming in through the folds in the worn out curtains, I preferred to read.

Four hours later the most enormous Russian-looking helicopter set down heavily on the frozen surface of the drop zone. An unshaven, heavyset man in a down suit covered in sponsors' badges stepped down from it, as if he had just come from another planet. I had never seen him before. I imagined the shock, for him, of landing back in this world after everything he had been through. We introduced ourselves and I was surprised. I am usually quite wary of these kinds of characters, setting themselves the wackiest challenges you can imagine with the sole aim of becoming famous. Most of the ones I have met have a huge share of egocentricity and a barely repressed inferiority complex. A fair proportion of them also fall into the border line category: an unstable psychiatric profile which, when pushed, strays towards the border zone between psychosis and reality. The latter are prone to the worst reactions when things get complicated. They are also capable of self-flagellation, which allows them to withstand great torment.

There are also great explorers who are more at ease on their own than in society and like the austerity of wide-open spaces. These ones love exploring the essential values of human existence through hard work and challenge. To return from this kind of combat takes you back to basics, allows you to appreciate the simple things in life and identify life's essential values.

I liked Mike a lot and was sure he belonged in the second category. I think he is the kind of person who does self-sufficiency better than living in society.

We had to set off. The one problem was the sled that didn't fit through the doors of the jet. We tried all sorts of angles but it was impossible. We would have to fold it in half. Mike was absolutely adamant he wasn't going to abandon it. It was as if we wanted to separate a snail from its shell. Touched by remorse, one of the pilots finally decided to dismantle the emergency exit, through which we had entered the cabin, and we finally managed to get the sled in the plane. Mike was happy and relieved. We could take off.

The return journey was very friendly. Mike had a phenomenal stock of foie gras and salmon packaged by one of his sponsors and friends, the famous Swiss caterer Rocha. We spiced up our journey with these heavenly foodstuffs washed down by the airline's champagne and travelled in high spirits. I also used the time to look at Mike's fingers, seeing as that's why I was there.

I felt his eyes boring into me as I took off his bandages and I was expecting the worst. His fingers were covered in phlyctenas, blisters typical of vascular stasis that leads to freezing of the tissues. The tips were slightly grey and some of the pads of the fingers were necrotic, yet overall it didn't seem like a hopeless case to me.

'I am inclined to think it is a stage three case,' I declared.

'What does that mean?' asked Mike.

'It means there is a risk we might have to amputate the end phalanges of three of your fingers.'

'So that means all is not lost?'

'It means you were right not to give in to your Soviet torturer.'

'You're sure they can be saved?'

'It's not out of the question. It's worth trying a shock treatment on them.'

Mike understood. Next stop: Chamonix.

Eight hours later we were in the department. I had called on ahead to make sure a room was set aside for our explorer. Dominique, one of the care assistants, who was very attached to the moral values uniting the staff of the unit, watched us with an amused look. It wasn't the first time I had brought back an extraterrestrial for her. Already under Mike's charm, she had lovingly prepared his room for him and slightly coyly showed him the door to the shower. What she didn't know was that Mike had been remorselessly scrubbed down by an enormous hairy female nurse with a scouring brush in the Siberian hospital and he was as pink as a baby!

I let him sort himself out in his new lodgings and went off to prescribe him some 'frostbite special'. This uses a new vasodilator that is much more powerful than standard treatments. After several years of perseverance and paperwork we had been given permission to use it as an experimental therapeutic protocol. It was a bit late in Mike's case but it was worth a try.

In the end, Mike kept all his fingers intact and set off on another new and completely bonkers challenge a few months later: the circumnavigation of the Arctic Circle. He did it, recounting the details in his book. I was engrossed as I turned the pages and read how he had survived his adventure and how much he had appreciated his stay with us. I was flabbergasted to learn that he described me as a guru!

I returned home, exhausted, but full of renewed vigour. Mike must have passed on some of his energy to me. To a certain extent I envied the fact that he was able to give himself the means to live out these kinds of experiences. I would treat myself to a good night's sleep to catch up on the jet lag my little Arctic escapade had given me, as it would be business as usual the following day.

BLOOD ON THE MOUNTAIN

· · · · · · · · ·

The winter had come back a few days ago. It was late afternoon and bitingly cold. I was on department duty with the big bumble-bee. That was what I called the new helicopter, which now shared the work of the Alouette whose long career would come to an end within the year. Its actual call name was Foxtrot. It is a big machine, twice as powerful and fast as the Alouette III. There are also twice as many seats inside. This means that in a single rotation you can take the whole team, the doctor, gear, dog and Grandma all at the same time. But it doesn't have the same atmosphere. It's compartmentalized: there's the pilot's cockpit up front and the rest of us in the back. When time is pressing, everyone can jump out as if on some kind of counter-terrorism mission.

While another team is in charge of the Mont Blanc range, we are required to look after the rest of the department. It was four in the afternoon and our work for the day seemed to have come to an end.

We had just been called to a heart attack victim in Notre-Dame-de-Bellecombe. The woman didn't survive despite our best efforts. It was an Englishwoman in her fifties, on holiday in the small ski station. She had been to see a cardiologist the day before, complaining of chest pains. The doctor hadn't found anything, the tests came back normal. He reassured his patient and let her continue with her family skiing holiday. She collapsed suddenly and without warning in front of her husband and daughter, who still didn't really understand what had happened.

I stayed in the helicopter for a few minutes, looking at the resuss bag and thinking. I had had enough of hearts that we couldn't get going again. And when, by chance, they did restart it was only to stop again a few days later, exhausted with zero brain activity.

Mountain rescues have a manic-depressive side to them. From one moment to the next, the context can change completely. You can go from a story with a happy ending and then plunge straight into a horror show.

My friend Ben, who does the same job as me and is eight years younger, had just been through a particularly black time. He had been on call three times and had had five deaths. But there was nothing he could have done. There had been a 300-metre fall and a rock avalanche down a couloir on the Goûter. A feeling of uselessness had been gnawing away at him for the past week. He was the master of intubation in crappy conditions, but sadly not organization and tidying things away. He had resuscitated countless patients over the past few years. His greatest success story, however, didn't happen while he was on duty. It happened one day when he was doing some personal training.

One winter's day, just as he was setting off up the first few metres of a small icefall near a *gîte* called the Crémerie des Glaciers, she fell at his feet … She was a nineteen-year-old girl. The shock of the fall caused her heart to stop beating. Ben immediately started chest compressions while her boyfriend went to call for help. By some kind of miracle, or perhaps thanks to the chest compressions, her heart started again. Two years later she started studying to be a nurse and came to Chamonix for her first internship, with Ben.

I felt a depressive phase creeping up on me. I discussed it with Bertrand, the duty doctor for the massif that day who was younger than me.

'It's really boring today, there's nothing to do. But you haven't stopped all day!' he complained.

'Yeah, and you haven't stopped stopping. Is that it?'

'If you like. How did your heart attack go?'

'The usual. We couldn't get it started again.'

While I was hoping to draw some energy from this conversation I realized that the job was going to wear me out. Even the actions, which I used to find exciting ten years ago, now left me a little world-weary. Pain relief, IV access, fluid resuscitation and intubation are the four pillars of emergency medicine in the mountains. The trick is to be able to do them in every imaginable situation. I had spent all these years learning how to do it. Now that I had examined the question from all angles and could be of use, I wanted to quit. What a waste!

Bertrand tried to reassure me, but I didn't have time to weigh things up as Robin, the duty rescue-fireman, called me.

'Manu, we're off again. Something near the Col des Saisies.'

'No? This late?'

'Yep and there's no dawdling. It'll be dark in an hour.'

'What are we doing?'

'A recce. There were shouts but we don't know where from. It's not going to be easy. We'll have to look.'

This was classic: we were just about to put the helicopter away and were getting ready to tidy things up. We had taken off our harnesses, put things on to charge ready for tomorrow and now we had to leave again. There are no hard and fast rules in this job.

The sun was deserting us and there was a gentle yet bone-chillingly Arctic breeze in the air. The winter hadn't packed its bags yet.

We had only been flying in the big bumble-bee for five minutes and all the north faces were already in shadow. We explored the valley floor, below the Pic de la Croix-Blanche, that was in the grasp of an icy anticyclone. Five pairs of eyes scoured the bushes and clumps of trees under rock bands that might have caused an accident. We were looking for ski tracks in this little visited off-piste area. Shouts had been heard from the hotel down below in the early afternoon but since then nothing. Someone with binoculars had spotted blood beneath a band of rock in the early evening.

The bumble-bee swung round, its nose pointing at isolated tracks that stopped right above a small cliff. They showed that a skier had jumped and, for once, the facts matched the description given by witnesses. What was the guy thinking? The drop below was at least thirty metres.

Daniel steadily dropped down the length of the rock wall. The EC 145 had an impressive effect on the ground below: the powder snow swirled around furiously in sprays of white and the branches of the ash trees were shaken bare. At the foot of the cliff, in the almost vertical debris cone just before the forest of scrub and brush, a man-sized bowl-shaped indentation in the snow marked the spot where someone had landed. Fifteen metres lower down there was a streak of blood next to a bush, but still nobody.

'Go down further, Daniel. The guy must have slid down and ended up in the bushes,' said Robin.

'Yeah, lower down … I see him!' shouted Mathias, the gendarme. I saw him, wrapped around the trunk of a tree.

'Looks like he's had it. With the fall he took,' said Daniel wearily.

There was blood everywhere. He must have been there for at least three hours.

Daniel had joined the team that year. Little by little he was learning about the daily tragedies that often make the job pretty unappealing. The bodies we pick up and take back, lifeless, to their families, not proud of ourselves and with the depressing feeling of not having been of any use or having arrived too late.

'Wait, I think he's moving!' cried out Daniel, desperately trying to get in closer.

'Don't get your hopes up. It's the turbulence from the helicopter making it look like he's moving,' replied Robin.

Mathias got the rigid plastic bag ready and checked the loop on his harness to be winched down to the body. It would be dark very soon, there was no time to lose. The helicopters are capable of flying at night and can even carry out relatively technical manoeuvres but winching a rescuer down to the tundra on the valley floor risked crashing the helicopter.

Alex, the mechanic, opened the large sliding door and checked the winch using the big remote control device. I was sure he got a real kick out of playing with the winch. It must have reminded him of his childhood. Like all boys, he must have spent whole days at a time playing with his toy crane.

The cold and the din of the engine swept into the cabin. Mathias clipped himself in and Alex used the hydraulic arm to send him off into space. I sat back as it was obviously going to be written up that I had been of no use today. Unconsciously, the stress of not knowing if the victim would need my help or not left my body. It was clear he was dead. It was awful to think of the slow agony he must have endured but a relief to realize his suffering was over. He was at peace now.

I was reminded of the feeling I used to get when I first started out. The selfish relief I felt on learning that the victim was dead and nothing more could be done. I was more worried about the help I was going to be able to give than the tragedy the person's death would be for their friends and relations. These days I'm more or less broken in and I no longer question my abilities. They are what they are. I surprise myself sometimes when I find I'm thinking about the psychological aspects surrounding the accidental deaths of the people we pick up and the moral considerations they provoke.

'Mathias to Fox.'

'Yeah, Mathias, we're listening,' answered Daniel.

'He's alive ...'

Stunned silence.

'Send down the doc and the chamois with the gear and stretcher,' Mathias added. Chamois was code for the rescue-fireman, Robin.

A rush of adrenaline brought me back to reality. I'd better get going. I barely had time to put my gloves and helmet on before Alex handed me the hook for lowering. Robin was already down with the stretcher.

'Hurry up, Manu. I won't be able to pick you up in half an hour. Let me know what's going on as soon as possible, so we can get out of here before nightfall,' warned Daniel.

Without replying I unplugged from the cabin system and clipped myself in, ready to be lowered down. It was clear it was going to end up in a scoop and run. I don't particularly like working like that. We would pick him up as he was, wrapping him up in the stretcher, without giving him anything and hoping he would hang on until we got to the hospital. It was far from satisfactory but there wasn't a better solution in this kind of situation. Finding ourselves without a helicopter would change the whole problem. If we were late and had to carry him down between the three of us, sinking into the powder snow with him as we went, we would finish him off.

Robin met me in a freezing tornado of powder snow. We only had twenty metres of slope to descend to reach the skier and it was already clear that, given the depth of the snow we were wading through, we could forget trying to carry him out. Mathias found himself beside the lifeless body, not knowing quite what to do. I had a quick look at his general condition and decided that if he wasn't dead, he was as good as. He already had one foot on the other side and it was only a matter of minutes before the rest of him joined it. His jaw was fractured in various places. He had lost so much blood that the gaping wounds on his face had stopped bleeding. He was on his last gasp; he had a glassy stare, his pupils completely dilated.

I wedged myself in the gap between two branches and tried to unpack my bag. It was extremely uncomfortable and the skier was lying in a position that defied the laws of anatomy.

He was completed twisted with his head downwards, covered in snow. I had almost given up hope. It was a hopeless case. The guy was dying, there was no point in getting upset. What could I do in thirty minutes, other than get him in the stretcher and evacuate him? I tried to find a pulse in his carotid artery. Nothing. I thought for a few seconds. Even if it was the most obvious solution, winching him up in his condition would finish him off. I couldn't do that. I had to give him one last chance.

Robin had managed, more or less, to attach electrodes to him and hook him up to the heart monitor. His heart was beating. All was not lost, there was still a glimmer of life left. I got my equipment out in the snow that was getting into everything. I tried, getting irritated, to pull my latex gloves on before starting work. But it was impossible: my hands were already freezing and the latex stuck to my skin and wouldn't budge. I gave up. We decided to get the skier on to the stretcher so that he was more or less horizontal and insulated from the snow. This was no mean feat. He was once again covered in snow, and just for good measure, it had got into the pouch where I kept my IV kit. I was giving up hope of getting anything done.

I went into autopilot mode, keeping my emotions out of the equation: oxygenate, inject, get fluids in, pain relief, sedate, intubation … I had plenty to be getting on with. But how? Get an IV-line in? His whole body was in spasm. I was working blind and tried to insert a catheter into the crook of his elbow. It was a waste of time, there was no blood left in his peripheral veins. I would have to try the central route. I was going to go straight for the sub-clavian vein and get a trocar under his left collarbone. I did them on a relatively regular basis in A&E and I was usually pretty successful. Robin helped me cut away the layers of his clothes. I would be able to insert the metal sheath in the trocar and guide the final catheter in. But I was too sure of myself and didn't prepare the last part properly. I had forgotten about the hole in the snow below me and my foot fell into it. The metal sheath slipped and the trocar came out of the vein, and there was no way I could reinsert it.

While I was doing this, Robin had got out the oxygen bottle and he too was fighting with the branches that had been complicating matters right from the start. Furious with myself for having lost the vein, I decided to intubate him without sedation. I had to attach him to the respirator and give him as much oxygen as possible for the moment. This turned out to be a disaster. His jaw was in pieces and the usual anatomical clues were shattered. I was in an impossible position.

A phone went off, it was the victim's. I heard Mathias answer and try to get information about his identity. His friend or family member at the other end had no idea what was going on. Mathias was finding it difficult to get out of a tricky situation. He wanted to get a bit more information about the victim but couldn't bring himself to lie. It was difficult to conceal the evidence and respect medical confidentiality. The phone's battery resolved the problem. The already somewhat disjointed conversation was cut off. We only knew that his name was Jarvis.

It was impossible to intubate him. If we were to have any kind of chance of saving him, we would have to properly sedate him. But that implied causing his blood pressure to fall even further and it was practically in his boots as it was. This is the eternal dilemma faced by emergency doctors with a patient who is slipping away. You have to give him or her as much oxygen as possible and to do that you have to intubate, which requires sedation. All the drugs currently available have side effects: they disrupt automatic breathing and dilate the peripheral blood vessels. When the patient is bleeding heavily, it is essential to fill them up beforehand in order to prevent the heart from stopping. I felt powerless.

Nevertheless, an idea started to form in my confused brain. I decided to put him to sleep with Ketamine, administered with an intramuscular injection. I gave him a good dose. If you're attempting the impossible, it may as well be effective. As if by miracle, two minutes later a vein appeared. Ketamine is one of the rare drugs to raise blood pressure with almost immediate effect. I nervously inserted a large orange catheter. Fortune was smiling on me once again. Without a second to lose, I emptied the contents of the hypertonic saline solution into Jarvis's veins. It was as if I was giving him a good litre of blood. I gave him an injection of celocurine and got to work with my laryngoscope.

'Manu, it looks like we're losing him,' said Mathias in a worried voice.

'Yeah, that's normal.'

I didn't say any more. I was concentrating on trying to find Jarvis's vocal cords among the clot of blood that had formed in the back of his throat. Robin did his best to help me and passed me the aspirator. But there was nothing doing. I wasn't set up correctly and he was doubled up on the stretcher in what couldn't have been a worse position. Unless I was just too crap.

'Shit! Shit! It's not working ... Bugger! Put the mask back on him, Robin.'

Robin did what I said, a little upset for me. That was it, I'd cracked; I'd given up. To top it all, Daniel, who had put the helicopter down a bit further down the valley, called us.

'Fox to Chamois.'

'Come in, Fox,' came back Robin.

'In ten minutes I won't be able to winch you.'

'Ok, we'll take him as he is. We don't have a choice,' I announced in frustration.

I wasn't proud of myself. In a last-ditch attempt, I abandoned the messy laryngoscope, ripped off the oxygen mask, grabbed a thinner intubation cannula and tried to pass it through his nostril. This sometimes works when you can't see anything. I pushed the probe, forcing it a little. I did my best to tilt his head so that his spine was correctly aligned. It worked and the tube slipped into place. I checked with the balloon and stethoscope. Victory! I heard the reassuring noise of air passing symmetrically into the bronchi. A warm feeling crept up my back. Never give up!

'Quick, we've just got time to hook him up!'

Robin attached the oxygen to the respirator while I taped down the cannula. Mathias quickly strapped Jarvis and the gear to the stretcher. In thirty seconds, I had replaced the empty IV with a full one and had added half a vial of fentanyl for the journey.

We heard the EC 145's engine starting up in the valley, impatient and concerned at having to do a winching as it was getting dark.

The helicopter arrived overhead. The powder snow flew up again in great eddies. Daniel turned on the powerful searchlight on the machine's belly, dazzling us below. Night had descended upon us like a black canopy. Clinging to Jarvis and his destiny, I was lifted up into space in the direction of the valley. It was already in darkness. The dynamics of the wind from the rotor hitting the wall of rock caused us to start spinning. As we climbed higher, the spinning got faster transforming us into some kind of flying whirligig. We hadn't had time to set up the anti-gyratory system that prevents this from happening. I resisted, jerking my head round like an ice skater, but it was getting unbearable. I didn't dare think about the abdominal hemodynamic strains this was putting on Jarvis, unless he had quite simply given up the ghost.

Above us, Alex had surely spotted the problem and signalled to Daniel to speed up and counteract the rotating. The spinning slowed down but the violent wind dragged us towards the back of the machine. The cable from which we were hanging could withstand massive forces. If I had forgotten that winching could be scary, this was a more than effective reminder. There was also my pack that was flapping like a flag in the wind and thumping me like I was a punching bag.

Jarvis and I ended up under the cockpit, on the back of the skid. Bringing a victim on board an EC 145 is more complicated than with the Alouette. The standard technique consists in arriving with your back to the skid, so that you can go over it without the stretcher getting caught underneath. You then have to swivel the stretcher round and go in feet first. This is manageable when the helicopter is hovering but things are very different when you are travelling at cruising speed. Alex pulled at me and the stretcher, while I heaved myself up using the side handle. The violent icy wind slamming into us was lifting up the stretcher like it was a sail. I was flattened against the cabin and was worried it would all go. I had no way of getting Daniel to slow down. Thinking he was doing what was right, he was heading as fast as he could to Chambéry to drop off the victim with multiple injuries in the resuscitation department. After a five-minute struggle, Jarvis was in the cabin and I flopped down with the cable between my legs. I moved the hood of the stretcher to look at Jarvis's eye. It was impossible to tell if he was still alive or not. The respirator was doing its job and that was all I could say. The heart monitor was too big and had been left below.

I was pleased to see a team waiting for us on the roof of the hospital in Chambéry. Three people in white uniforms seemed to be happy to chat away until the rotor blades came to a stop. I couldn't tell if they were porters, nursing assistants or doctors. I broke the atmosphere slightly as I got off the helicopter.

'My patient really is dying here.'

The three guys perked up and we ran towards the resuss room. It felt like an episode of *ER*!

'Ok. Ready to lift?'

'Ready,' the three sidekicks replied almost in chorus.

'Lift.'

A strap was caught. Classic. Two bits of equipment fell on the ground. A nurse, who was a little older than the three others, started whingeing. Just in case there wasn't enough tension in the room already.

'Ready to put him down?'

'Ready.'

'Down.'

The on-call anaesthetist took over. He noted down, in a very professional manner and without saying a word, all the information I blurted out to him about the patient in no particular order.

Jarvis was in a terrible state and we hadn't even had time to wipe his face. The nurses undressing him must have thought we had done a pretty sloppy job. In their haste as they removed his left sleeve, the IV that I had such trouble getting in to him was ripped off. I sighed. We plugged in the wires and his pressure was back up to 9, his heart was beating … The anaesthetist got ready to insert a line deep into his femoral vein. Poor Jarvis, if only he knew what we were putting him through! But why did he jump that cliff?

I collected my equipment and, filled with a sense of hope, left Jarvis in the hands of the care team. Would he make a complete recovery?

We headed back by night to the Col des Saisies to pick up Mathias and Robin who were waiting for us near the lights of a small village. I told them Jarvis was still alive, he had got over the first hurdle. There was a slim chance he would survive. Everything depended on what the scans revealed.

It was eight in the evening when we got back to the deserted Drop Zone in Chamonix. The only light was in the hangar, to put the bumble-bee away. We unloaded the helicopter. My resuss bag was a complete mess and it would take me another hour to sort it out.

The winter season was drawing to an end and the team was ready to drop. Hoards of tourists had passed through our hands and as usual the A&E department had been full to bursting. As we did every year, we told ourselves that's the last time, never again. I'm handing in my stethoscope. This is a mug's game. As with every year, there weren't any beds left in the hospital. Also, just like every other year, we were shouted at by people with very minor injuries who were in a hurry and wanted to jump the queue. They were there on holiday, not to injure themselves. It was ruining our health and we had had some pretty frightening moments. And, just like all the other times, it was over and we forgot about it until the summer season.

It was the end of the week and the start of spring, the atmosphere was subdued. We had tried to prepare Khando for her departure but it was hopeless. She was digging her heels in. She wanted to stay. There were heart-rending farewells from all the family on the station platform in Bellegarde.

I was taking her to Paris but couldn't go with her to the airport the following morning as I was on duty. I had to return to Chamonix the same evening. Céline and I were extremely annoyed that we couldn't go with her as far as the aeroplane. But there was no way we were going to hand her over to Marie-Jeanne, who had suggested she help. Our relationship had not improved.

We arrived in Paris and went to Gilles's house. I had recently met him in Chamonix and we knew each other a little. He was looking after a young Nepalese teacher from a school in Dolpo who was visiting France. When we told him our story, he offered to accompany Khando himself, and I immediately felt I could trust him.

Khando looked very sad and started crying. I had explained to her time and time again that it wasn't the end, that if she didn't go now, as her visa was running out, she would never be able to come back. In the end, I just had to leave her with Gilles and his wife who would do their best to reassure her.

The following morning, at the hospital, my mobile went off just as I was getting ready to sew up a trainee chef's finger that he had cut to the bone. It was Gilles. He handed the phone to Khando in frustration. She had thrown a tantrum. She had decided she wasn't going to leave. I gave her as gentle a talking to as I could manage while trying to show a modicum of authority. She came round in the end. I said goodbye to her, but it was all that I could do to put the phone down.

I needed a few moments to recover my composure. The trainee chef gave me a sympathetic look.

3

SUMMER

· · · · · · · · · ·

GERVASUTTI PILLAR: FRIDAY

• • • • • • • • •

Summer in Chamonix, or Death Valley, as some of the British tabloids would have it. The valley is brimming with brash youngsters waddling their way through a minefield of objective dangers. From the helicopter you see them all over the valley, hanging from rusty old pitons and roped up like strings of sausages. Every time I fly over the massif on busy days I am amazed that there are so few accidents, given the number of climbers and walkers there are per square metre.

Olivier was waiting, fuming, at the ticket counter of the Aiguille du Midi cable car station. He was furious with Rob. It was always the same; he was incapable of arriving on time. Rob ran up to him sweating and rosy-cheeked, with his flies undone. His pack wasn't properly closed and dangled miserably from his back, strewing half his belongings on the ground behind him.

'Rob, you've dropped a glove. Come on, hurry up! Here's your ticket.'

'Yeah, it took me three hours to park! It's incredible, you even have to pay to park now!'

'Oh for Christ's sake ...' moaned Olivier.

Rob was a complete mess, but a good bloke nonetheless. He spent his entire life in a daydream. He could never say no and as a result he was always in over his head.

Olivier had met him in the Verdon five years before. He had found Rob quite irritating at first, with his veneration for Chouinard gear which he considered collectors' items. It had become an obsession and he had a whole cupboard full of the stuff. In fact, Rob was more of an obsessive than a collector and he would, without fail, launch into some interminable explanation or other to which Olivier would listen politely while thinking about something else. Yet Olivier found him fun to climb with. He was rather endearing and very considerate of others and for Olivier this, more than anything else, made up for his other faults.

They got to know each other better during a trip to the Ahaggar Mountains. Rob had been seized by a sudden passion for photography on their expedition to the Sahara. He had fallen in love with an old Leica and took photos of everything with it. He would spend hours at a time lying in the sand fine-tuning it and setting up shots. Some people had found it irritating but it entertained Olivier to watch Rob lost in his own little world, amazed by everything and anything.

The lift silently started up for the Plan de l'Aiguille. Rob continued packing his bag, elbowing all those around him, while Olivier chatted with Max and Dod and checked their gear.

They had been planning to climb the Gervasutti Pillar for some time but had never quite managed to get to it, as either the weather was bad or one of them couldn't make it. But it was a joint project and they had promised themselves they would do the route together. The conditions had been good the whole week and they had a window of opportunity left for the climb before the bad weather came in at the weekend. It was now or never.

The Gervasutti Pillar on Mont Blanc du Tacul is no small undertaking. Guidebooks describe it as a two-day route, though strong teams now often do it in a day. The lads were feeling fit and had done some good circuits at Fontainebleau. Olivier had been training by cycling round Paris and Max had climbed a 7c. They were all counting on him to do the crux sections. In any case, they had no intention of having to bivouac. Bivouacs were for has-beens. They were modern mountaineers who climbed fast and lightweight!

According to the guidebook it was quite straightforward: they would sleep at the Cosmiques hut Thursday night, do the Gervasutti Pillar on Friday and go back to the hut the same evening. They would have a little bit left over at night if there were delays. The bad weather wasn't due in until Saturday night, so they had some leeway …

Two o'clock in the morning. Four specks of light shuffled below the Col du Midi towards the Rognon.

'Hey, lads. We've got a problem.'

Despite the lack of light, Olivier had noticed that something was wrong. Rob had the look of someone who had screwed up and you could expect just about anything from him.

Rob was in bad way. The night at 3,500 metres had shaken him up. He had been sick twice in the night and couldn't sleep. By midnight he wanted to take a sleeping pill and now he was wasted.

'Come on then, out with it,' said Olivier.

'I've forgotten my harness.'

'Oh, well done! Now what do we do? Any great ideas?'

'Erm, I guess I'll have to leave you here. You can climb as a three. In any case, I'm not feeling great ...'

'No, that's just stupid. You can climb with a sling, we'll make a harness for you. And, looking at your face, I don't think you're going to be doing any leading. You can be Max's second.'

'Oh, thanks. I'll kiss goodbye to my nuts now, shall I?'

They had difficulty leaving the hut and it was later than planned. But this was a small problem, given the crush at breakfast. In the bag room there were people and things everywhere. There were small ones and big ones, those doing the TVB (traverse of the Vallée Blanche) who had got up at two in the morning to make sure they didn't miss the last lift at six in the evening, and those leaving to do the MBVT (Mont Blanc via the Tacul) were too tired to think. There were women crying because they had two left shoes and a Spaniard who couldn't find his friend. The latter must have already left, thinking his mate was looking for him outside.

'Oh shit, wait. Wait! My crampon's come off.'

'Rob! For Christ's sake!'

Olivier was starting to think that today wasn't the day for all this. Then again, as the night faded, they could make out the shape of the Gervasutti Pillar.

Six-thirty. Max was trying to find the route up the wall of rock.

'Oi! Max. You at the stance yet? We're freezing down here!' Olivier shouted up, sounding irritated.

As it was dark, Max had taken a guess at where to start, not having stood back and studied the route, especially not the first pitch. Now he wasn't sure if he was even on route. And the rock was wet. He had kept his big boots on and it was hardly a piece of cake. He was finding it really tough and this was supposed to be grade 4+! This was a far cry from the red circuit at Milly-la-Forêt! Some time earlier he had come across an old peg that had reassured him, but since then there had been nothing else for at least the past fifteen metres. He was in a bit of a precarious position. His left foot was resting delicately on a small flat hold covered in lichen, his left hand was pulling on a tiny slanting crack, while his right foot was probably on the only decent hold he had and his right hand fumbled around desperately trying to find a hold.

'Fucking hell, what am I doing? This should be a piece of piss!' he snarled out loud.

After a few minutes' hesitation, he straightened his left leg, trying to find a nubbin of rock to make the next move. Anyway, he had to try something as the muscles in his thigh were progressively tightening. Murderous thoughts came into his head as he listened to the others complaining about the cold. This was a really bad start to the pillar. If he ever got hold of the bastard who equipped this route ... And still there wasn't the slightest peg in sight. His headtorch was of no use to him any more and the moment had come in the dawn light when you didn't know if it was still night-time or if the day had begun. In short, he couldn't see a bloody thing.

With the help of a bit of acrobatics, Max managed to slip a friend into the tiny crack he was using for his left hand. He attached a quickdraw to it. And before clipping the rope in, he gave it a little tug, more out of habit than conviction, to make sure the friend was in properly. I wouldn't even clip my mother-in-law to that, he thought.

'Slack! Shit, give me slack!' he bellowed, pulling on the tight rope.

The worst of it was that the others had no idea of the shit he was in. The pressure mounted. Suddenly a burst of adrenaline prompted him to get out of the position that had become untenable. Max decided to go for it and move his left foot up on to a wretched little crimp. He tried to put his foot as close as possible to his buttock. He was also aware of the fact that he probably wouldn't be able to push up on his leg with his big bag and the friction on the rope. What an idiot! Why didn't I put my rock shoes on?

He took a good thirty seconds to focus, breathing hard like a bull. He stood up heavily and let out a stifled cry. His left hand tightened, one of his nails broke and his whole body tightened in the same movement. The aim was to grab what looked like a spike higher up.

But it was no good. There was a sickening noise and he fell away with the lump of rock. Max's hand scrabbled away at the rock in a final attempt to hold on but the weight of his pack had got the better of him. The quickdraws and friends he was wearing on his harness produced a spray of sparks as they scraped on the granite. He fell five metres and miraculously found himself suspended from the pathetic friend he had just placed.

'Max, are you ok? Maxou?' screamed Olivier, to whom the jolt had come as a surprise.

'Yeah. Yeah, I'm fine …'

He was winded and his body had gone limp. He stayed there for five minutes, feeling pretty wobbly. Here was someone who climbed grade 7 every weekend and he had spent an hour on some crummy grade 4 pitch! It was pathetic.

In the meantime, the dawn had taken on its crimson veil, chasing the dark away. Ten metres to the right, a crack line sat taunting him. What an idiot! It was so obvious now. He was almost ashamed of himself.

It took a further two hours for all of them to reach the top of the first section, where they came face to face with three Poles who were calmly eating breakfast outside their bivouac tent.

THE DEAD GUY'S NOT DEAD

· · · · · · · · ·

I had had a pretty relaxed day the day before. Cécile had dropped Pierrot off at a friend's birthday party, Alix was playing at Aline's and we had a quiet day pottering around the house. Seeing as the weather wasn't good enough to go climbing, Céline set about making jam. Through the window, as the hours passed, I saw the pots lining up on the kitchen counter. For my part, I was determined to finish the terrace. I had started it over a month earlier but had made little progress: the pile of sand sat imperiously in front of the covered play area and the stack of salmon-pink paving slabs hadn't got any smaller.

I set off the following morning untroubled. It had rained a large part of the night and a glance up at the mountains led me to think that I could expect a relatively quiet morning at the DZ. The sky was completely socked in and there must have been ninety kilometre an hour winds on the Aiguille du Midi. I could take my time, swing by the hospital, have a cup of coffee and answer my emails while I was at it.

By eleven o'clock at the DZ everyone was going about their own business. While three rescuers were sprawled on the sofa watching a daft TV programme, three others were putting the world to rights over their umpteenth cups of coffee. Down below two rescuers fiddled with the gas supply to the Paillardet winch and I was sorting out my bag. I took out all the broken phials, bits of sticking plaster and empty packs of transparent film that were all over the place.

Bob came in for his Sunday morning visit and he was looking well. Bob was our mascot. He was eighty-one years old and still going strong. He had been one of the valley's first rescuers and even figured in the *Uncle Paul Stories* that I used to read in *Spirou Magazine*. I adored the *Uncle Paul Stories* when I was a kid. There was one about the perilous rescue Bob undertook in the middle of a storm to evacuate ten people who were trapped in the old Mer de Glace cable car. Bob had kept a faded copy of the magazine. The cartoon strip showed the rescuer – Bob – balancing on the roof of the cable car helping the terrified passengers. The helicopter team had extremely skilfully winched him down to it. I liked to tease him by calling him Bob Sinclar, after the French DJ.

He got his attack in first as he entered the hangar, asking me, 'And how is the eminent faculty professor this morning?'

'Hi, Bob.'

'Things ground to a halt, have they, doc?'

'Yep. It's good to take it easy from time to time. And how's the blood pressure?'

Bob seemed to be living on borrowed time, as he had had a few health problems and he had been given a pretty pessimistic prognosis. Bob laughed when he recounted all his problems but he had been putting up with them for seven years and wasn't about to give up yet. To listen to him, the worst of them was his failing memory, about which he complained incessantly. Much to the disappointment of the members of the Chamonix Mountain Rescue Association, of which he had been the President, Bob preferred to resign for fear of making mistakes with the funds. His thing was now trout fishing and when he wasn't out with his mate Jacques, Bob could always be found at the DZ as he liked to know what was going on.

That morning for the fun of it I took his blood pressure.

A tear appeared in the blanket of clouds in the early afternoon and there wasn't a single rescue to disturb our idleness until three o'clock. Jules, the duty pilot, got a call from Cordial.

'Yeah ... Ok, but at what altitude? The Col de la Brenva. And we don't know any more? Right, we'll have a look. Hang on, I'm just looking out the window ... Yeah, it looks ok. We'd better get going.'

'Are we off?' somebody asked.

'On your feet everyone. We're going to have a look on the Col de la Brenva. The storm hit some folk up there and we've got to collect them,' explained Jules.

It needed something like this to get them moving.

Ten minutes later I was flying with them. I had politely been asked to join them, as one of the exhausted climbers was unconscious. As usual, I didn't know any more. Was it heart failure, was he hypothermic, the living dead? It wasn't a very useful report.

At 4,000 metres the helicopter was buffeted around and it felt like the cabin was taking a real beating. At certain times, it was as if there was no air beneath us and the drops were enough to bring up yesterday's breakfast. The bad weather was still here. I watched Jules battling with the joystick, and as the machine plummeted and climbed I thought I was going to bring up my lunchtime sandwich as well. We could make out the ground through the clouds. But where were we? It had to be the Col de la Brenva.

'Fuck, this is some wind! This isn't going to be plain sailing! I'm not going to be able to stay for long,' announced the pilot.

All of a sudden a guy appeared out of nowhere and ran towards us waving his hands.

'Langlois, get out and see what that guy wants! I'll try to come round again and pick you up,' ordered Jules.

Yan opened the sliding door and put his head out to see where the back of the helicopter and the skid were in relation to the snow. The Alouette was leaping around like a little goat.

Jules was starting to get irritated.

'Go on, jump. I can't hold it much longer.'

Langlois jumped. I stayed in the helicopter. We beat a hasty retreat from the col and dived down towards the Petit Plateau. It felt a bit better having a bit more space around us.

Ten minutes later Langlois radio-ed up to us.

'You've got to come and pick up two people. There's one guy in a snowhole who looks dead, an Englishman, and the other one doesn't look much better and he's in another hole … A Frenchman, apparently.'

The howling wind was causing interference.

'Ok, I'll take one at a time,' Jules replied nervously. Before quickly adding, 'Manu will pick them up for you. We'll send him down for the first and come back for the other one.'

And the fun and games started all over again. It felt like we were flying in a washing machine. I opened the door and jumped out to give Langlois a hand. We loaded the first victim up and I jumped into the helicopter. The Frenchman looked totally rigid. Yan shut the door and we dived off again.

I looked at the climber: his body was stiff and he had his elbows and wrists folded over his face. His legs were like wood and were completely frozen. But there was a slight doubt in the back of my mind and to assuage my conscience I swept the snow off his face. His cheeks were frozen and his features contorted, yet I thought I could see a glimmer in his eyes, under the corneas veiled in ice. I tried to waken him but had difficulty moving his arms. It was then that the incredible happened. The dead guy wasn't all that dead after all: he was moving!

'Jules, the guy's not dead! I'm telling you!'

'So what do I do? Am I taking him to the morgue or the hospital?' asked Jules.

'Hang on a minute.'

I took his temperature with the tympanic thermometer. Twenty-five degrees. This was incredible. I tried to attach my mini heart monitor to his chest to see what his heart rate was. I managed to pull away the top of his frozen Gore-Tex jacket, which together with all the layers underneath was clamped to him like a straitjacket. The vibrations from the helicopter caused massive interference and I couldn't get anything from the monitor. Ventricular fibrillation, sinus bradycardia? It was impossible to tell. I sat there powerless, wondering if I should give him heart massage or not. I opted for the latter in the end and, in any case, we were already at the hospital. We had landed without me even noticing. The door opened and there was a gurney waiting for the patient.

We unloaded the deep-frozen mountaineer, unceremoniously sliding him on to the metal surface of the trolley. Before I even had time to recover the heart monitor, I saw my guy being taken away by the nurses. I almost had to fight to retrieve my equipment.

The helicopter took off again with a deafening roar. The stunned onlookers watched us, wondering what kind of disaster we were off to. I prepared myself psychologically for the next victim. Would he be another of the living dead?

There was still a gap in the clouds above the Tacul. Langlois was yelling into the radio.

'Come in, Dragon, this is Langlois.'

'This is Dragon. Go ahead, Langlois.'

'Are you coming?'

'Yep. With you in seven minutes. How's it looking?'

'I can see the Aiguille du Midi from where I am. You should be all right but the wind's really gusting. We can't hang around.'

'How's the second guy?'

'He's completely stiff but alive. Have you got Manu with you?'

'Affirmative.'

'He's gonna have to look at him pretty quick. It's weird. He's squirming all over the place. We had trouble tying him up.'

Was this a joke? This was a pretty unusual situation, as I generally preferred to go down to the patient and prepare him or her for evacuation. But this was what one might call a case of *force majeure*. In a quarter of an hour the clouds would come in again and we were going to look stupid stuck out high and dry at 4,000 metres with a case of hypothermia on our hands!

The Col de la Brenva came and went a few feet below the helicopter. We were like a bottle of Orangina bobbing about in a storm.

Jules managed to set us down as best he could a few metres from Langlois. The door opened, I grabbed the guy and dragged him into the cabin like a sack of potatoes. The whole machine was shaking and it was too risky to pick up Langlois as well. We made a quick getaway, diving down the slope to make the most of the ground effect. The top of the Aiguille de Saussure passed between the helicopter's skids and the machine stabilized itself. This allowed me to get a look at our convulsing Englishman.

He didn't look like anything described in the books and it felt like I was dealing with one of those street artists who do robotics. He was as stiff as a windup toy and wouldn't stop wriggling. He was moving so much I couldn't take his pulse. I tried to slip the oxygen mask over his face, it was an intuitive gesture that had never failed before. He struggled, doing his best to push my hands away. There wasn't a single sound coming from his mouth and his vacant and fearful expression made him look like a zombie.

The helicopter headed into the mist, its blades spinning, and a breath of warm air hit my face.

'Jules, can you turn down the heating, please?'

'You don't want me to warm you up?'

'Yes I do, but not like that.'

I was thinking of the story of the girl who died on the Aiguille du Midi in similar conditions. Utterly exhausted and frozen to the bone after having made a winter ascent somewhere, she managed to get to the top station of the Aiguille du Midi. Thinking they were helping, the lifties sat her in front of the stove to warm up. She went into cardiac arrest a few minutes later and they had no idea why. Heat causes the peripheral blood vessels to dilate, yet that creates a massive drop in blood pressure causing the heart to fail.

I would have liked to have taken his temperature with my tympanic thermometer but it was in the bottom of my bag and we would be at the hospital by the time I had found it. Better to wait until we got there.

It was about time we landed. The guy was wriggling around as if he was trying to get out of a straitjacket. He was really worrying me. The door opened and I shoved him out. He seemed to calm down a bit.

The resuss trolley was waiting for us outside the double doors to the hospital. The department was busy. I ran into the nurses' office to drop off my bag, shouting out all the usual instructions as I went.

'Get him hooked up to a monitor. We need to see what we're dealing with. And he's not very warm either.'

'Shall we cut off his clothes?' asked a nursing assistant, brandishing a pair of scissors.

I had always found it difficult to wreck mountain equipment that cost a fortune.

'Try and attach the electrodes down his front so that we can monitor him as we undress him,' I suggested.

'Ok, let's get him on to a hospital trolley and get started.'

He fell on to his left side as we moved him from the emergency stretcher to the hospital stretcher and the step under the trolley shook him up again. This was obviously not the thing to do, as he started flailing around once more as if he was having convulsions.

At that moment Big Chief, who had been told about the odd goings on, turned up. A quick glance was all he needed.

'Let's go. It looks to me like your chap here is going to go into cardiac arrest.'

It was the tone to take and he knew how to put the pressure on! The small team of staff – that was us – got moving and it was as if someone had given a hefty kick to an anthill. A few minutes later the Englishman was hooked up to a monitor, intubated and having a cardiac massage. A thermometer inserted into his rectum confirmed his 25°C hypothermia. Things were not looking good for him. Defibrillation was out of the question until his core temperature was above at least 30°C.

All cardiologists say that a heart can only start again once it is warmed up. That is the point of having a machine to provide extracorporeal circulation. Unfortunately, not everyone has one in his or her garage. Not only are they expensive but they also require a specialist team to run them twenty-four hours a day. We used to have one knocking about somewhere in the old hospital but as it was only ever used two or three times a year the anaesthetists weren't really up to speed. Currently, only large hospitals with heart surgery units are able to provide this service. As we didn't have one, Big Chief had developed some very simple active internal heating techniques. They have been described in great detail in medical textbooks by authors who have, obviously, talked them up a great deal. Yet, as is often the case, it is easier in theory than in practice. These procedures consist in warming a patient up through circulating hot liquids through all available internal spaces. The peritoneal cavity, pleural cavity, bladder and stomach are all good for circulating saline, which has been pre-heated to 38°C, using tubes temporarily inserted through membrane walls.

The story of the two Englishmen who tried to climb Mont Blanc via the Goûter could have been quite run-of-the-mill. The storm came in as they reached the final hump and it was a white-out. They were 200 metres from their objective and decided to try their luck. There was no one else on the summit, apart from a couple of Frenchmen who were also caught out in the bad weather. The French climbers were a couple of locals. One of them was a customs officer in Chamonix. The four of them found themselves in the same tricky situation and one team decided to follow the other. The Englishmen followed the Frenchmen down towards the Col de la Brenva where the slope slackens off. They were wandering through gusts of hail and the wind had filled the track in with snow while lines of sastrugi conspired to throw them off route. As they reached the first depression, which they identified as the Col de la Brenva, the storm was at its peak. As was their exhaustion.

The Frenchmen dug a snowhole and the Englishmen did the same, twenty metres away. As is always the case, one of the Frenchmen lasted longer than the other. And the same went for the Brits as well. In total that made two men fighting for their lives and two others who had sat back, waiting for death.

According to the heart monitor, all was going well for the first of the two patients: thirty-seven beats a minute. Our frozen man was waking up! We removed his mountaineering clothes and covered him with a heated blanket. We set up an IV-line injecting his veins with 38 degree isotonic saline solution and now everybody watched him with compassion. Everyone stood round him, ready to pounce in case the thought of going into ventricular fibrillation should enter his head. Everything was ready for a huge resuscitation attempt. But following the after drop, his core temperature started to climb steadily.

The term 'after drop' is used at every possible opportunity at conferences and refers to a somewhat poorly understood phenomenon: when the core temperature of a hypothermia victim you are warming up drops. Paradoxically, instead of their temperature rising, it drops more. Several different, and rather involved, explanations have been put forward. For the time being, the most rational one rests on the transportation of massive amounts of cold blood from the extremities to the core. This is always a delicate situation, as the heart is very unstable at this stage. It doesn't take much for it to start racing and pass into fibrillation, which is effectively heart failure. You would think you could easily get it started again with a small jolt from a defibrillator. But the problem is that the temperature of the heart must be up to 30 degrees if it is to stand a chance of restarting. While you are waiting for this, heart massage is the only alternative. This makes the odds of survival rather limited in a small hospital that doesn't have an extracorporeal circulation machine.

This is undoubtedly how the Englishman died in the room next door. He wasn't as lucky as his companion in misfortune. He had obviously gone into cardiac arrest as we brought him in and even though we tried to warm him up as quickly as possible and to keep the massage time down, he remained impervious to all the techniques used by Big Chief.

All the information was there: two hypothermic climbers had been picked up in the same condition and from the same place, and they both had temperatures of just 25°C. Three hours later one of them was asking us the time and wanted to go home and the other one was dead. I was incapable of giving a decent explanation.

What had pushed one to survive but had sent the other one irreversibly the other way? From now on, how could I not have serious doubts about the diagnoses of death we had made in the mountains? After all, what defines death? How could I be certain a climber was really dead when he had been found frozen stiff in a hole in the snow but with no obvious signs of injury? What was to say his heart hadn't simply progressively slowed down at the same steady rate as the organic functions it served? What was there to prove that his brain wasn't unharmed? Why couldn't we expect his heart to restart if we warmed him up properly?

As our eminent colleague Emsley Smith put it, 'No death from hypothermia can be declared as such until the patient has been warmed up.' This saying at least had the value of inciting us to review our working methods. The message spread slowly: in the mountains, a patient is not pronounced dead until we have established a clear medical history. From now on, when they have the slightest doubt, rescuers try to have a doctor on hand to check the tympanic temperature and detect the first signs of cardiac instability. The logistics allowing the patient to be taken straight to a unit with an extracorporeal circulation machine are far from in place. So we have to make do with ad hoc health care measures.

I went home, lost in thought. The day's events had prompted much discussion among us all. The two hypothermia victims had added even more grist to our mills, as Big Chief with his fondness for reworking old expressions would say. We would have to reassess our procedures, organize ourselves and rack our brains. In fact, our comments always came back to the same conclusion and that was that the only way to improve our treatment of these kinds of cases was to treat more of them!

I had another look up at the top of the Tacul, hidden behind a seething mess of clouds buffeted by the violent winds that continued to speed them along. It couldn't be much fun up there in this weather.

The hypothermia that hangs over climbers now hounds me in my sleep. The 'white death' doesn't always take those she wants and I have never thought we were equal before her. I was able to prove this, to my cost. Sooner or later, if you push things too far, hypothermia will burn your fingers. And that's what happened to me a few years ago in the Himalaya.

WHITE DEATH

· · · · · · · · ·

I was coming to the end of a three-month stay in the upper Dolpo region where I had been lucky enough to work as a guide and doctor during the filming of Eric Valli's Oscar-nominated *Himalaya*.

I had made the most of my time off during the long weeks spent at 4,000 metres to scale all the local mountains. I often climbed the wild peaks alone, the difficulties being relatively moderate. Some had probably only ever previously been climbed by a few adventurous locals.

Thanks to these excursions I was quite well acclimatized to the cold and the altitude. Living with the Dolpo people had helped me identify with them and, like them, I no longer needed a down jacket to keep me warm in the evenings. Like them I now ate tsampa, yak yogurt and yak butter tea. I was also now capable of carrying increasingly heavy loads and crossing mountain passes at 5,000 metres in trainers. I was even trying to compete with the porter we had nicknamed TGV owing to the speed with which he ran up mountain paths. I was hardly about to give him a thrashing but it was something to aim for. Perhaps I would have liked to have been born in Dolpo?

I gradually climbed increasingly tricky routes. All on my own, obviously, and with no rope or climbing gear. At the most, my bag contained a water bottle, a few energy bars and some barley flour pancakes I picked up at breakfast.

I had set my heart on climbing a rather difficult looking wall of rock. I found myself cornered at an altitude of around 5,500 metres on a crumbly band of rock. I down-climbed the fifty or so metres of crumbling unstable rock. A little voice in my head was telling me to give up and go back down to the valley, not to let my pride get the better of me. But it was all in vain, I was on a complete high and was blinded by my own arrogance.

I had taken missing out on the summit of Everest by just a few dozen metres very badly. It was my excessive caution that had caused me to turn back and I had never fully got over the sense of disappointment and regret. I had taken this hugely important decision, weighing up a pointless victory against a headlong dive into the abyss, into my very consciousness and soul. This choice often shows in the vacant expressions on the faces of dead climbers we pick up at the foot of climbs. With a feeling of guilt and perhaps trying to deceive myself, I sometimes try to recreate in their expressions the final instants of their combat, the ultimate decision that was the worst choice of their lives.

Thankfully, as I stood alone on Everest's south summit without bottled oxygen, there were a few neurones still working in the right side of my brain, its logical and analytical hemisphere, the 'conservative' part that gives the orders. At 8,700 metres, even though I only had 300 metres to go along a corniced ridge to the summit, I had obeyed like some kind of automaton. Such was my state of utter physical and mental exhaustion, that I might never have come down alive if I had made it to the top. Full of a wealth of experience, my subconscious had taken the decision for me.

After Everest I swore to myself that if I started something I would always finish it. Mountains, personal projects, I would never again take something on without seeing it through to the end. This kind of all or nothing attitude became my philosophy in everyday life.

This choice reappeared in Dolpo … On the crumbling rock face, it was my left brain that won the day. I had never been a particularly expert rock climber but I had been climbing since my eighteenth birthday. I had climbed on all kinds of terrain imaginable, from the most featureless slabs to the most crumbly cliffs. The rock I was on now was not unknown to me. It was a kind of red and grey limestone that looked like the most eroded sections of the Verdon gorge, and God knows I had climbed some bad rock in my time!

I had just down-climbed the same part of the face twice and was in a bad mood. I had calmed down by the third attempt and decided to get up it whatever it took. This moderate but loose climb was requiring all my powers of concentration. I moved from loose flake to loose flake, spreading my weight as much as possible and using up to three wobbly holds at a time. I would have liked to have stayed agile and lightweight on the unstable holds but I was short of breath and my moves sluggish. Shaking and completely pumped, I finished up the last few metres of climbing with a hysterical cry, which thankfully nobody heard. By following some old snow leopard tracks along a dead-end snow ramp, I finally found an escape route. I reached the summit happy but a bit shaken up.

This, however, was not enough to calm my ardour. As I walked back down to the stunning Phoxundu lake, I couldn't take my eyes off a snowy 6,000-metre peak that pointed up above the camp where Cécile had joined me, and from where the two of us would go trekking.

The mountain had the delightful name of Kanjirolawe and was part of the Kanjiroba chain. Obviously, without a permit it would be impossible to climb it under the nose of Kalipati, the liaison officer who had been with us since the filming started. Kalipati was the only one, of the three liaison officers we had been assigned, who was still with us. The film's director thought he would go mad if he had to put up with them for the entire duration of the filming. Fortunately, the first one had packed his bags soon after arriving, claiming to have a variety of acute mountain sickness symptoms, which I had no trouble in treating with complete professionalism. As for the second one, I had given him an antiseptic known to turn your urine red and he had preferred to return to Kathmandu pretty sharpish to get tests done.

As for Kalipati, he had stayed as he was a naturally jolly sort and fared particularly well at altitude. Unlike all the other liaison officers I have known, he genuinely liked his work and took part in festivities with a certain gusto. We became friends. It is quite unusual to get on well with LOs. Most of them are parasitic, two-faced, penny-pinching pen-pushers from the Tourism Ministry, who are totally incompetent in the mountains. You can easily spot them at expedition base camps, as they are the ones who leave their tents with a piece of terry-towelling – and it's always the same kind! – wrapped round their heads like a turban. They quickly become hate figures when the expedition learns it has to pay them over a thousand dollars, feed them and look after them for the entire length of the trip. What's more, everyone knows that a large part of the money goes into the pockets of a few well-off members of the Nepalese administration, while our porters are weighed down by our excess baggage for a few hundred rupees a day. Kalipati knew a few basic words in French that he proudly claimed to have learned when he, or so he said, had studied seismology in the dim and distant past in Paris's Jussieu university. We got into the habit of exchanging language lessons in our free time.

I was torn between the desire to climb the mountain and my misgivings about having to deceive Kalipati. Nevertheless, I was fiercely opposed to the pre-emption that certain countries, such as Nepal, have over their mountains. I don't think they belong to them, so much so that I felt I was in my rights to climb them. I had discreetly been up other peaks in the area and I thought I would be able to go about climbing Kanjiro-lawe in the same manner. What you can't see, won't hurt you...

I left Ringmo very early, telling Cécile I'd be back the same evening. Just enough time to do a trifling little 6,000-metre peak! I felt really strong and was going great guns. At no stage did the thought cross my mind that the face might give me the slightest problem, and I had neither crampons nor ice axe in my pack. I had equipped myself with a telescopic trekking pole, which only half worked, and a dirty pair of scrappy old overtrousers. I had kept my boxers on though, and they would surely keep me warm, at least where they didn't have holes. I had observed the face from various different points in the valley and it was there for the taking. I would claim it as I had claimed the others, alone and in silent anonymity.

I set a good pace, and was light on my feet, almost ecstatic, making my way up the innumerable mounds of polished rocks spat out by the now dry stream that drained off the immense snow slope of the southeast face. The face appeared to flatten out the nearer I got and started to look quite easy. My blood was up and as it pulsed warmly through my veins, it cleansed my mind of any reservations. I was flooded with feelings of happiness and it felt like I was a kid again. Three hours later, however, my mood changed as the slope steepened. I had climbed up the snow slope and found myself precariously balanced on an almost vertical slab, weighing up the dangers, which in my euphoria I had previously failed to spot. To reach the ridgeline leading to a final small rock pillar, I risked taking a 700-metre fall.

Retracing my steps was out of the question: there was no way I could walk down the steps I had kicked in the snow with my boots. In any case, as the snow got harder with the cold and the altitude the final section had been virtually rock hard and I had felt less and less purchase under my feet. The rock in front of me looked preferable and, besides, I didn't really have a choice. It was no more solid than the other rock I had come up against over the past few months: cracked limestone flakes and gravel. I had thought there would be an easy ridge awaiting me after the exhausting climb up the previous fifty metres but I felt the colour drain from my face as it revealed its true nature to me. To the right was a blue-tinged chasm covered in powder snow that would slide at the slightest touch, while to the left lay snow as hard as ice that had melted and refrozen. There was no way I could cut steps through it. I would just have to crawl! Luckily, my body was still willing. I wasn't hungry and I felt as if I was only at 3,000 metres; the altitude wasn't bothering me at all. An hour later, on the slopes below the pillar, I found myself sinking into deep snow as it collapsed under my feet. It got into my jacket and under my modest layer of outer clothing.

There wasn't a single decent hold on the steep mixed pillar standing between me and the summit ridge. The rock was completely loose and the snow rotten. I exhausted myself as I did my utmost to gain more ground than I was losing, hauling myself miserably from one patch of névé to another.

I don't remember what time it was when I reached the summit but the sun was still high in the sky and I was filled with a sense of joy. It had only taken me a morning to climb 2,000 metres at an altitude of 6,000 metres: I couldn't be in that bad shape! Plus, I still had enough time left to walk off the immense pyramid via the ridge on the other side.

This was before I had discovered the nasty surprise that was waiting for me. I drank a few mouthfuls from my bottle, finished off my chapattis, and headed over to the other side of the snowy summit dome. In the space of a minute I realized my predicament. The final 300 metres of the ridge, which I couldn't see from below, actually formed a compact plug of ice dropping away to a slope that was over 60 degrees! A small cluster of séracs halfway down the face formed a slight shelf and the slope below seemed to ease off down to the snowy ridge that led to the bottom. But down to the séracs I wasn't going to get much purchase with my Contagrip soles!

I had a choice between the toboggan of death or the ski jump from hell …

I walked round the mushroom of snow on the summit and realized I was trapped, a bit like being on an iceberg in the middle of the ocean. Down-climbing the crumbling pillar seemed pretty dicey and I certainly didn't see myself back-tracking down the 700 metres I had just climbed without crampons. It would have been suicide. I went round in circles for over an hour wondering what to do. Anxiety was creeping up on me, giving me an unpleasant feeling in the pit of my stomach.

A final alternative presented itself: descend the first 100 metres of the steep rocky face separating the two main ridges and pick up the ridge I wanted a little further down, where the slope eased off and the ice seemed to turn into snow. I set off down-climbing, in the knowledge that nothing could be more unpredictable than a slide down the slope. Alarm bells were going off in my head. I was in a phase of absolute concentration: each step was absolutely critical and there was no margin for error.

The descent wasn't very extreme to begin with but I sensed this wasn't going to last. I saw icy gullies starting from the base of the summit platform that I was clinging to. I wasn't going to get far without crampons as I simply couldn't afford to set foot on hard ice. But I was hoping to lose enough height to reach the ridge at around the level of the séracs. Armed with a pointed dagger of rock in each hand and putting my toes on small rocks imprisoned in the ice, I set off on the most delicate traverse of my life. The series of icy runnels were separated by vertiginous lines of rock, which thankfully gave me enough support to be able to relax a bit. I had been hopelessly deceiving myself: the closer I got to my life-saving ridge, the steeper the slope I was on became. I shuddered as I set off on the final twenty metres.

'Shit! What a fucking idiot!' I shouted out loud, not feeling any stronger or braver for it. I felt really stupid. I had been in this sort of situation so many times before in my life that I wondered how I could have showed such a complete lack of good sense this time! When I was a kid my best friend and I got ourselves into similar scrapes trying to do a tour of the neighbourhood's roofs. We jumped from one section of guttering to another for the thrill of it, to the utter despair of our mothers who dreaded each day's new challenges. Thirty years later here was the same kid clutching a couple of lumps of flint, his muscles so tense they were fit to burst, trembling with fear and crawling over ice gullies with his eyes fixed on a paltry bit of ridge.

When I was close enough I threw myself at it like a man possessed, death seemingly snapping at my heels. My two bits of rock tumbled over the precipice and I felt strangely naked but not unhappy at having made it. I had won some utterly stupid game! I chanced a look over the other side, unsure of what I was going to find. I had ended up right on top of the intermediate platform formed by the press of séracs dividing the slope in half. I was saved! Or at least that was my initial impression ...

My second impression was an altogether different one: I was in fact trapped like a rat on an ice floe. I still had fifty metres of ice to descend to reach the snowy ridge I thought I had already found. Fifty metres of 60-degree ice would have been a mere formality if I had been wearing crampons. But it was hard grey ice and my footwear was hardly designed for this kind of terrain. Whatever happened, I would finish up on my arse and there was a pretty slim chance of me ending up sitting astride the adjacent ridge. To my right there was what must have been a 1,000-metre drop, while the one to my left was a little shorter, maybe 950 metres.

I paced up and down my tiny island of ice. I had tried everything: climbing back up the dome, searching for a line on the west face and even trying to find a way through a tunnel in the séracs, which seemed to open at the bottom. I had ended up dangling with my legs in space, floundering like a fish out of water.

Then icy black night fell, its chilly breath piercing me through and through. This wasn't funny at all. It brought me back to my senses. I awoke from my torpor realizing what would happen to me. The faces frozen with frost of those we hadn't been able to save flashed through my mind. Fit and healthy men frozen solid in the ice. You're going to have to fight this, I told myself.

A quick calculation gave me a glimpse of what I would have to endure during the longest night of my life. At the lake by the village of Ringmo, 2,000 metres below, we had recorded night-time temperatures of −10°C. I knew only too well about the temperature lapse rate: it falls by .85 of a degree per 100 metres climbed, to which you also have to add the wind chill factor. So I could expect to have to put up with temperatures of around −35°C, and that was if I was out of the wind. This, of course, wasn't the case, as I was perched virtually on top of a mountain.

Yet I had no intention of dying, I wasn't meant to go like this. Cécile was down below and my kids were waiting for me in France. I was going to put up a fight. I was going to have a think, and then put up a fight!

I prepared myself for a long and uncertain sleepless night. I watched the sun reddening behind the mountains and told myself it was very beautiful but very unhelpful. Giving up at a moment like this wouldn't be nice! The Phoxundu lake far below frowned up at me, it waters the gloomiest icy black imaginable. The Mediterranean blue that made it look so heavenly during the day was just a memory. No more birds or insects, there was just the wind to answer me. I was bombarded by the great questions in life: Who am I? Where am I going? What the hell am I doing here? There was the same response to all of them: what an idiot.

'Cooee, anyone there?'

This was the joke I liked to play when I found myself climbing at my absolute limit, eight metres above the last rusty peg. There's nothing to say you can't make a joke just because you're inches from death! This usually relaxes me and sometimes gets a laugh out of my friends but this time it didn't even make me smile.

I was aware of the Earth's immensity as it stretched out beyond the horizon and I thought that, relatively speaking, the bottom of the mountain wasn't very far away after all. And that reassured me a little.

I stamped both my feet the whole night long. It was time to put into practice all the advice I had given in specialist magazines and to people who had asked my opinion before setting off. I remembered Alain Bombard, a doctor who had taken to the ocean to prove his theories on survival at sea. He drifted across the ocean in a rubber dinghy for weeks on end. I was carrying out the same experiment, except that I wasn't prepared for it and I might not survive.

I dug myself a hole with my feet. I didn't want to use my hands as I wanted to keep my Monsieur Bricolage suede sheepskin gloves dry, otherwise my fingers would freeze. However, nothing could change the fact that I was sitting on a suspended balcony of rock-hard snow. Even using my boots, I couldn't get more than a few centimetres through the hard carapace of ice. As I'm a glass is half full kind of man, it occurred to me that, at the very least, my efforts would keep me awake. My repeated digging would keep my core temperature up and the time it took wasn't important. The time I could spend huddled in my hollow, keeping my muscles working, would perhaps stave off severe hypothermia. Then it was just a question of how long the batteries would last, as Big Chief would say.

I had a limited amount of time but I was incapable of evaluating it rationally. My hero, Einstein, would have certainly had an explanation as to why I was so out of kilter. I had been banging away at the ice for hours, or so it felt. But the harder I dug the harder the ground got. I had cut away just enough for my buttocks and they too were starting to feel pretty rigid.

I focused all my effort into trying to combat the cold which was progressively taking hold of my body. It was slowly coming up from the ground and I was steadily losing a few tenths of a degree at a time through shaking, which was also draining my precious energy reserves. I redoubled my effort at digging and breathed down my collar to warm up my chest. I had folded my already numb fingers into the palms of my hand to try and make the most of the final few calories left in my circulatory system, which I sketched in my head from memories of anatomy classes.

I had pulled my hat down to my neck and zipped up my Gore-Tex jacket, the one remaining piece of protective clothing of any use in the environment in which I found myself trapped. The funniest thing was that I found a tensioner cable for a moped at the bottom of my pack. There really was a bit of everything in there. This was a good illustration of how relaxed life was in the austere Dolpo region during those long months. I wrapped the cable around me like a belt to keep the clothes next to my skin. We commonly tell people that a small layer of air between your skin and your clothes acts as insulation. Well, it's not true! Don't ask me why, but that's just the way it is and I know because I have tested it. The cable kept me warm.

I daren't look at my watch, knowing how slowly time passes in these kinds of situations. And that was an understatement. When I thought it must have been past three o'clock in the morning, I risked taking a look. It looked like the night was waning, as if the sun had done its trip around the globe and was on its way back. Wrong. My watch said ten-twenty-five. It was sickening. I was already shaking a worrying amount as soon as I stopped digging and I had only been struggling for a couple of hours. This really knocked me for six. I decided to cheer myself up a bit by turning my headtorch on. It's silly how much good surrounding yourself with a little halo of light will do! Two hours later, exhausted, I tried out my hollow. Hunching up my shoulders, I managed to protect myself, more or less, from the piercing wind. Yet the fact I had stopped moving caused a rapid drop in my temperature and I was shaking uncontrollably, meaning I had dropped below the 35-degree mark. The struggle wasn't going to be fun.

An hour later one of the first symptoms of severe hypothermia – the imaginary friend – appeared. He was a nice enough bloke but I couldn't tell you what he looked like. I had a kind of split personality and I remembered thinking that my soul should break away from my body. My curious companion was giving me advice: 'Breath into your shirt, swing your arms around … No, don't just give up! Come on, fight it! Get up! Get back to work, you're gonna die!'

I felt an icy white death creeping up on me. It was starting to feel as if it would be nicer to give in to it than carry on fighting. In the end, dying like this might not be as bad as all that … I was so numb that my already oxygen-starved brain cells were starting to go into hibernation. I thought about the Canadian salamander, which although deep-frozen to –10°C, thaws out and comes back to life in the spring. I really would have liked a bit of antifreeze in my cells too. In the meantime though, I was a hair's breadth from giving up.

All of a sudden my whole life came down to the hole in which I had plonked my bum and which I had not very successfully hacked out of the ice. Nothing seemed more important to me than my kids, my wife and those closest to me. It was life and that was it. I was going through a stage in survival that everyone should experience at least once in their life. That night the precariousness of existence would reveal its true value to me. The minor hassles of daily life and the pathetic arguments that get people upset, political skirmishes and spats about wearing religious clothing and symbols at school, the state of the stock market or the value of the Euro;

all of these things paled into insignificance compared with the void that surrounded me. I was going to die, it was as simple as that.

I took a photo of myself with the little Nikon that had never left my side for the past few years. It was a ridiculous thing to do but left me with the hope of living long enough to be able to let out a little forced laugh looking at it in years to come. It also helped to pass a few minutes in this interminable night of anguish.

After a long series of psychological struggles and hallucinatory jousts, dawn finally started to break. My hopes slowly returned. I felt like I was on the brink of an epileptic fit as I couldn't make a single move without shaking uncontrollably. My energy reserves were utterly exhausted and I had undoubtedly also started to attack my protein stocks. My body was eating itself. By some kind of miracle neither my fingers nor my toes were frozen and I was proud of myself. Yet my problems were in no way resolved. I was still in front of a wall. An impassable wall of ice. And no one was going to come and rescue me from the top of my roost, especially seeing as only Cécile knew where I was.

So I rooted around in my pack, in the half-hearted hope that it might contain something useful that I hadn't spotted before. A bit of rope, an ice screw, a magic lamp maybe? There was nothing left other than a minuscule first aid kit in which I found a pair of folding scissors. They were ancient and a bit rusty and I must have salvaged them from some old expedition kit. However, they were pointy and quite robust. I looked at the scissors then back at the slope, telling myself that this was probably my last chance.

Time is what I had, so I set about cutting steps the old-fashioned way. I thought about the pioneering ice climbers who hacked out notches in the ice for their feet. I calmly crouched down and meticulously imitated them. Metre by pathetic metre, with one leg dangling, clinging to the ice, I made my way down the slope that had held me in its icy hell. I scarcely remember how I got down the rest of the face, as it seemed positively trifling compared with what I had been through up till then. I was ecstatic to have survived, as if this had been *the* great ordeal of my life.

GERVASUTTI PILLAR: THE STORM

• • • • • • • • •

'For fuck's sake! Rob, what are you doing? Climb!'

Rob was exhausted.

They had finally all managed to reach the top of the rock climbing section of the route. It was eight o'clock at night and their hands were caked in blood. Max had found the last few pitches really hard going but couldn't understand why. A combination of the weight of his pack, the altitude and the route had slowed him down. To make matters worse, he had had to down-climb twice as the rope had been caught on spikes of granite. Rob was incapable of climbing up to unhook the rope without a belay. The worst of it was waiting for Olivier and Dod. They were freezing cold after three-quarters of an hour of not moving. A few big clouds had appeared over their heads and the gusts of wind were getting more and more violent in the two corridors to the side of them. Even the Alpine choughs were finding it difficult. At one point, they were comforted by the thought that the hardest part of the climb was out of the way. But they were mistaken, as Max quickly found out. The unstable mixed ground that followed seemed to go on forever. Olivier and Dod had preferred to untie at first, only to tie on again later, as the climbing got too difficult. This also slowed them down.

It was eleven o'clock at night. What they had thought would take them an hour had actually taken three hours. The rock was now covered in snow. Rob was completely drained. He had used up a lot of energy following Max and had been in over-drive for the past few hours.

'Rob, what the hell are you doing?' asked Max impatiently.

'I had to put a layer on and get out my headtorch. I couldn't see a thing,' explained Rob, wearily.

'It doesn't take two hours to put a jacket on! Now I've got to put extra clothes on, as I'm freezing waiting for you.'

'Oh, come on.'

'Look, we've got to get moving, we can't be far from the top … Where are the others?'

'Dunno … The last time I saw them was on the mixed stuff.'

Max and Rob just had to wait, huddling up against a mound of rotten rock. The snow had been whipping their faces for a good ten minutes before the first clap of thunder crashed behind the pillar of rock to their right. Rob, his teeth chattering, almost swallowed his tongue. Max saw his companion's eyes nearly pop out of their sockets as if he'd just seen the devil himself.

'Shit! Max, did you see that?'

'No, what?'

'Christ, Max, stop it! I hate thunder. We've got to get out of here. Are we near the top?'

Max tried to unfold the photocopy of the page in the guide-book that was already soaking wet and torn to bits.

'I have no idea. It's never ending. We've got to cross a kind of saddle and head right, on to the north face for at least 250 metres to reach a ramp …'

'Think you can find it in the dark?' asked Rob.

'Do you think I know? I'm not sure I can go on either.'

Crash, a second clap of thunder. And now it was hailing too. Rob did his best to brush off the hailstones that had already settled on the top of his pack.

'Ol-iv-i-er! Do-oo-od!' bellowed Max into the darkness.

Silence.

'For God's sake, what the hell are they doing?'

Max and Rob huddled together. They were getting seriously cold as the falling snow stuck to the rock, gradually turning the route to ice.

Suddenly a shout rang out.

'Maaaxou!'

It was definitely the two others. But Max didn't immediately react. Like Rob, he had let a cold lethargy creep up on him. It was only the second shout that made him jump.

'That's them, Rob! They're here, I can hear them.'

Olivier and Dod finally reached them, frozen to the bone, their faces haggard. Dod had a shattered cheekbone from slipping on a sheet of rotten ice and Olivier hadn't been able to feel his fingertips for over an hour.

'We went wrong at the first gendarme … We thought the route went behind … It was crap. We ended up on completely the wrong side. The bottom of the slab is as slippery as fuck with just a crappy old peg … We had to go back the way we'd come! By then the ledges were full of hailstones … It was bloody dodgy! Touch and go!'

Olivier was so shattered he had trouble explaining what had happened. They had finally picked up the normal route again, despite Dod's grumbling.

Dod had totally freaked out.

'Now we're really in the shit! We can't see anything, in the middle of a fucking thunder storm! And where did this shitty weather come from? I thought it was supposed to be good up to Sunday.'

The weather had indeed worsened and the conditions had become icy. They sat in silence, trapped, not knowing what to do. It was gone midnight and no one could take it all in. The wind had died down a little, but only so that it could snow more heavily.

Max was aware of the fact that the three others were counting on him to get them going again. They would have to try and find the fabled exit ramp higher up. Rob had already slipped into a far from restful sleep. He had none of the energy of the day before. Max rallied a bit and suddenly leapt up, shaking himself like a dog and whooping like a legionnaire.

'Fuck it. We're not going to stay here and freeze to death like a bunch of idiots. We've got to get out of this hole.'

'Max, we can't see a thing, it's three in the morning. It'll be better tomorrow morning. Try to get some sleep,' said Olivier.

There was another clap of thunder, less than 100 metres away. Each time it made the other two jump, as if waking from a nightmare. It was unbearable; it had been going like this for over three hours. You might read a hundred accounts of them in books, but nothing can express the utter terror you experience during a storm in the mountains. Will-o'-the-wisps, bolts of lightning, fireballs, they were all there, especially in Rob's already fuddled mind. The icy cold had frozen him to the bone. He tried to comfort himself by remembering the image of Professor Calculus blown off his feet by a bolt of lightning in the middle of the drawing room of Marlinspike Hall in *Tin Tin and the Seven Crystal Balls*. It was very funny as a cartoon strip ... He also thought about his collection of Chouinard Camalots and stoppers neatly arranged in the cupboard in his room back home in a wealthy suburb of Paris.

Max decided to try and make a break for it.

'Rob, pay out the rope. I'm going to see what we can do.'

Rob had difficulty understanding what Max was saying to him. It was windy and dark, why go on? He watched the rope slithering out limply in front of him and wondered what it was for.

'Rob! Slack!'

The rope squirmed. It was a snake. That's what it was, a poisonous snake! Vermin!

'Slack, Rob. The rope's caught. Slack.'

Just in case, Rob gave the tangle of rope a kick.

Five minutes later Max came back.

'Shit. I can't see a thing.'

He threw himself on the ground and started to groan as he hit his hands against his thighs in an effort to get the blood flowing back into them.

'I can't feel my feet any more.'

A few hours later a semblance of dawn broke. The wind was still furiously slamming into the abrupt walls of rock on either side of the Gervasutti Pillar. There were fewer showers of hail but it was still intensely cold. Max had fallen asleep, his arms buried in his jacket. He didn't have the heart to take off the coils of rope round his chest. Rob looked like he was petrified under a carapace of ice. His eyebrows had turned white and it looked like they were stuck to his small pair of glasses, which had frosted over. Their two companions were hunched together, shivering, only half conscious. There was a strange atmosphere, as if the inseparable group of friends had decided to stick it out and await their fate together.

It was around midday that Rob finally lost the plot completely. Three rumbles of thunder came one after another and lightning crashed a few metres away from him. He jumped and stood up like a zombie.

'It's a chopper! Hey guys, can you hear the chopper?'

Nobody could hear anything except the thunder that was getting louder. The other three would have liked to have heard the helicopter but, even as they strained to listen, they couldn't make out a single sound. Then Rob moved forward, without the others being able to make the slightest movement, and fell into space …

It was Sunday and Olivier's family was the first to worry. Three days without news. It wasn't like him not to let them know what he was doing, especially not if he was heading off into the mountains.

Several phone calls from Paris were enough to raise the alarm with a PGHM rescue team. Two rescuers checked the car park at the cable car station for cars matching the descriptions given and a call was made to the Cosmiques hut. It wasn't difficult to reconstruct the missing climbers' route.

'Hello, Cosmiques hut.'

Marianne was manning the phone that morning as she sorted out invoices. It looked like being a quiet day. The bad weather meant most of the climbers had cancelled their bookings, while the few who hadn't gone down the day before were playing Liar's Dice.

'Yeah, hi Marianne. It's Lionel.'

'Hey, Yoyo, how's it going?'

'Fine thanks, you?'

'I'm taking it easy. Making the most of the bad weather to have a look at the accounts while Christian's making a flan.'

'Listen, Marianne, we're trying to find four climbers from Paris who were supposed to do the Gervasutti Pillar. Ring any bells?'

It was as if Christian's flan had just clattered to the floor. Of course it was ringing bells! We could often cross-check the information Marianne provided with our own when we were looking for someone. Yet so many people used the hut that she could hardly be expected to remember one person more than another. Nevertheless, she clearly remembered Rob's face. She had watched him that evening, looking a bit lost, trying to find his friends' table in the dining room. She was filled with an unsettling sensation and described what the man, who had to be Rob and who the others were teasing remorselessly, had been wearing to Lionel. She was a bit embarrassed when she realized she couldn't describe the gear Rob's friends had on. She told Lionel she hadn't seen them come back and the bad weather had come in much quicker than had been forecast on the Tacul. They must have got stuck somewhere near the top. Christian gave her a puzzled look as she put down the receiver, a far-off expression on her face.

Furious gusts of hail had battered the windows of the hut the whole night long and the good weather wasn't forecast until the beginning of the week. Marianne had another look out of the window at the summit of the Tacul. It was completely socked in, the top of the east face wreathed in thick clouds.

The depression had come in from the northwest, more quickly than forecast and catching out all those on east-facing climbs. It must have been hell on the Gervasutti. She could make out the waves of hail and snow washing down the upper section of the pillar and shivered.

MARVELS OF MODERN TECHNOLOGY

•••••••••

The weather hadn't been too bad in the valley the day before and we spent it running around picking up people, so I had decided to take it easy. We had got rid of the kids, as they were staying with their grandparents, Arthur and Lucette, for a short social rehabilitation course in the Vercors! With that, I was able to do a night shift at A&E and Cécile could look after her B&B guests. Then we made the most of the good weather and had a laidback day climbing in the Aiguilles Rouges. The climbing here is not as difficult, committing or as high as the neighbouring range. There are no glaciers and no enormous face climbs and the routes often have quite a rustic feel with stunning views of Mont Blanc.

That Monday morning back at work was chilly for the summer. I was at the DZ for the week of the 14 July, which looked like being tough. Legions of cars with foreign number plates were backing up at the level crossing for the Montenvers railway. They were back, they were here and it was going to be a big one! I learned that there were already four people missing on the Gervasutti and we were waiting for the weather to improve to start a search.

As I was wiping the windscreen with the sorry remains of a scraper, the radio I had left on the car seat started to bray. Often it isn't anything to panic about and just because it's making noise, there's not necessarily any work for the medic. Sometimes it's the helicopter on a technical flight, while other times it's someone telling his mate where he's left the keys to his 4x4! But this time it sounded like a proper rescue. I vaguely heard someone talking about Le Planet or a name like that. The only problem was that there were at least three villages in the range with that name!

I got a move on as it looked like this was one for me, a trauma of some kind.

The take-off woke me up. It's hard listening to the shriek of the helicopter engine when you haven't had your morning coffee.

We were already over the Col du Tricot, looking for a man who hadn't managed to finish his message. He was using a mobile and it was probably France Telecom, given that it kept cutting out all the time. The guy didn't sound good and he only had time to jabber the names of the chalets near where he fell.

'Right have a look, see if you can't spot something,' said Yaz, the pilot.

I couldn't see a thing as my eyes were still half asleep, and that's not counting the myopia.

'There! I see something. Eleven o'clock. Down below,' cried Marco.

Yaz dived down and we saw someone at the bottom of an avalanche couloir. The picture became clearer the closer we got.

'Have you seen the guy? It looks like there's a pool of blood next to him. He must have gone off the top with the slide,' said Marco.

'Wow! That's at least 200 metres!' added Yaz as he sorted out his approach to come in at the right height.

The injured man started to move about when he heard the helicopter. Watching him from above, he looked like a kind of savage running around on all fours. Ten metres below we spotted a broken snowshoe, which the machine's rotor blades sent spinning. There was something about the guy that bothered me but I couldn't put my finger on it. The helicopter dropped us off with the stretcher then flew away. I looked in the direction of our man and I still couldn't work out what didn't look right. Judging by his slightly stunned look, Marco was just as puzzled as I was.

'Do you think there's something odd about his head?' he asked.

'I can't say I can see his head.'

'Excuse me, sir. Are you ok?'

Suddenly, as I made my way up to him, I realized what was wrong.

What we thought was his face was in fact a figment of our imaginations. From far off, he looked shaggy, his greying hair long and tangled, especially at the sides. Yet on his head there was nothing! His scalp had been almost totally ripped off and hung down at the front like a curtain, only held on by a few centimetres of skin. It covered his face down to his chin with only his naked scalp on top, as if he had a tonsure. Thankfully, we couldn't see his brain!

'He looks like that monk from the Chaussée-aux-moines ad,' said Marco, a little queasily.

'Watch out, he's dripping all over the place,' I said, adding a more serious tone.

The man was waving his arms in our direction, as if he needed to feel a human touch. I asked him to calm down, explaining that we were going to put everything back where it belonged. After having slipped on a pair of surgical gloves, I lifted up the bloody flap of skin that was hanging down and placed it on the naked skull. It made a rather unappealing plopping noise.

We wrapped a length of crepe bandage round his head, maharajah-style, and headed to Chamonix hospital at the double.

We dropped off our 'wild man from the woods' at the hospital to have his scalp, or what was left of it, sewn back on. It looked like a good hour's work and a few reels of propylene thread would be needed.

People say a lot of unkind things about mobile phones. Some people can't bear to be parted from the stupid, yet at the same time, useful things. They take them with them on walks in the mountains, thinking that at the slightest fart a guardian angel will sweep down to their rescue.

We have noticed the impact mobile phones have had on our job over the past few years. One day we were called three times for the same rescue, which was a little irritating.

A man had waddled off a walking path. He was with his family, from the north of France, and even the best of them hardly had their sea legs. Our man, wanting to show off in front of his wife's family, managed to get his paws tangled in a root. He rolled about ten metres through thorns which, as we know, are always strategically well-placed. His sister-in-law,

Josette, was better at getting her mobile out than giving first aid and feverishly dialled the emergency services before even finding out if he was hurt. Cordial sent it to us and asked us to have a look.

We duly took off immediately only to turn round again thirty seconds later when, seeing as the victim assured her he was ok, Josette cancelled the call out. However, on clambering out of his ravine, the man discovered that he had indeed turned his ankle and was having difficulty walking. Now not daring to dial 15 for fear of getting an earful, our Josette called mountain rescue direct.

'Hello, is that the mountain rescuers?' she asked. 'My brother-in-law can't walk. In the end it would probably be better if the red helicopter could come and pick him up.'

'Is this for the same person?' asked the gendarme at the other end.

'Yes, it's us!'

'Ok, we'll send the helicopter,' he replied a little coldly. 'Where exactly are you?'

'Er … On a path. In the mountains.'

'Yep, I'd got that much. Which path precisely?'

'Well … We left the red cable car that goes up to the Pic du Midi about an hour ago. And now we're on a path that goes to the other end.'

It took the gendarme a good ten minutes to find the approximate place in question. And that was exactly the same amount of time it had taken us to get out of the helicopter, unpack the gear and flop down on the sofa in front of some crappy American series. We had missed the beginning but thought we could catch the end. Then the phone rang.

At the other end the gendarme was a bit embarrassed about bothering us again and said in an exasperated voice:

'Right, lads. Remember the rescue that was cancelled? You've got to go back. Turns out he's done his ankle in.'

There were a few groans but we just had to lump it.

'Where are they?' asked Henri.

'They had a bit of bother explaining. But from their description they're on the Grand Balcon Nord around about the Aiguille de l'M or below the Nantillons glacier. I thought they were in the Pyrenees when they started telling me about the Pic du Midi! The guy in question has got a khaki waxed jacket and brown trousers. So that shouldn't be difficult to spot! They've confused the mountains with a hunting trip.'

The same team set off once again. Christian, at the controls, hovered a while before gaining height, to check out the female tourists sunning themselves on the banks of the Arveyron. Then he started on the usual dance up over the larches: right a bit and then left, trying to find the thermals to carry the machine up to the Nantillons glacier. Once there, we had to look. Given the number of crossed arms and waving anoraks on the Balcon Nord you'd have thought there were wounded all over the place. The hikers saying hello to the helicopter are legion and finding the actual victim among them is not easy. In fact, we often head for the ones not waving their arms, which seems to work every time.

After ten minutes of to-ing and fro-ing we spotted a group that seemed to match the description. We would have liked to have landed but one of their number didn't seem to want us to. He was waving his yellow jacket and didn't look very happy.

'What does that bloody nuisance want? He's standing in the one place I can land!' shouted Christian.

Each time the pilot came in to land the same nutter came out again, as if he was trying to stop a tank. We finally touched down with just a single skid thirty metres below and Henri jumped out to go and see what all the fuss was about.

Three minutes later he called in.

'Come in, Dragon, this is Henri.'

'Go ahead, Henri.'

'The guy doesn't want rescuing because he thinks it'll cost a fortune and he'd prefer to carry his brother-in-law down on his back. I told him to calm down, it wouldn't cost a thing and not to mix up mountain rescue with the tourist information centre next time.'

'What are you doing now?' asked Christian.

'Apparently it's not that bad. I put a splint on him and now I'm calling you back to pick him up.'

'Ok.'

The problem with mobiles is that sometimes they might save the life of someone who could never afford a radio, while other times they are used for trifling matters. Soon enough we'll get called out before the accident has even happened!

With no other rescues to go to, we returned to the DZ. As I put my bag down on the torn stretcher we used for resting survivors, I heard yelping. A naturally curious type, I stuck my head out of the doorway.

'Hello, fatso!'

The big doggy didn't move a whisker, proving that gendarmerie Alsatians are not the kinds of dogs to roll over and wriggle their bellies to show how pleased they are to see you.

He was tied up at the entrance to the building and looked quite calm. His thick fur stuck out over his collar, and he was definitely the top dog. Avalanche dogs are big beasts. Trained for search and rescue, they are also used as guard dogs. Over the years I have spent several hours patching up the damage caused by these cuddly bow-wows: a hand here, a cheek there and even a nose.

I looked at him and he in turn stared at me, a suspicious gleam in his eye. Even though he was tied up, I gave him a smile to keep us on friendly terms, not going anywhere near him. All the more so, because I didn't know his name and am wary of all dogs, a hang-up from childhood. When I was a kid, adults said I had an affinity with animals, right up until the day one jumped on me. That certainly calmed me down. Now I give them a wide berth. And a few months before, while I was walking along a pavement in Iquique in Chile in shorts, a filthy mutt, who waited for me to walk past so as to surprise me from behind, clamped its jaws into my calf. He got what was coming to him. I had a weighty 800-page tome, together with a full litre and a half bottle, in my beach bag and before I knew what I was doing, I had swung it at him. I whacked it in a great circular movement, leaving him lying stunned on the paving stone. That one was for all the others, too!

Inside the medical office, I battled with a ray of sun coming through the window and hitting me right between the eyes, stopping me from being able to read the computer screen. I had a huge pile of records to catch up with and wanted to make the most of the morning lull to enter them into the database we used each year for statistical purposes.

It is surprising just how much the creation of such a service – the medicalization of mountain rescues – depends on many things but not an effort from governing bodies. 'Show us that you can be of some use and we will see what we can do' seemed to be the attitude. It's true to say that if you've never been suspended over the void, your face covered in blood and screaming in pain, you won't know how useful a mountain rescue doctor can be. If you've never dislocated a shoulder or broken a femur on the ski fields, you won't know the benefits of morphine. But there we are, not everyone goes on holiday to the mountains, certainly not those churning out the literature behind our health care system.

In reality, the medicalization of mountain rescues was born out of the desire of a small group of individuals keen to work in an exciting area of medicine, rather than any health care or political need. If we hadn't been there a few years ago, would there have been any other unconventional medics willing to take up the cause? It took fifteen years for the essential nature of the profession to be recognized. Although it seems obvious these days to have a doctor on rescue missions, we had to move mountains for this to be accepted. I sometimes still ask myself if we are the only ones who think this is obvious. We sometimes get the unpleasant sensation that the money might stop coming altogether if a minister doesn't crack his head open on a fir tree!

In the beginning, we had to plead for funding. Although this was never enough, we carried on working, mainly because we felt passionate about it. The hospital's director, under pressure from Big Chief, had created several short-term contract placements that weren't terribly rewarding but we took them all the same. Chamonix hospital was already in the firing line from the departmental health authority, which wanted to get rid of it as soon as possible. And anything that might justify its presence on the health care map was not welcome.

I was turning the issue over in my mind, asking myself where we would be if we hadn't taken the bull by the horns, when I saw a woman I didn't know walk past the door. Come to think of it, I had seen her once or twice before with one of the gendarmes. She must have been his girlfriend. She nodded to me and carried on towards the garden, and I went back to my files with all the professional conscientiousness of a good civil servant.

A few minutes later my concentration was broken by a little plaintive shout. I looked up but didn't hear anything else and returned to my statistics. A few moments later I heard the same far-off voice again, a smidgeon louder this time.

'Is anyone there? Er, help!'

Silence. Obviously the job was really getting to me, I was seeing and hearing danger everywhere! But the voice came again.

'Please, somebody help me!'

I stuck my head round the door and was taken aback by what I saw. It was pure *Candid Camera* and I was tempted to go and fetch mine but decided that wouldn't be very gallant on my part.

The woman had obviously wanted to give the hound a pat on the head as she went past, but the dog, who weighed not far off forty kilos, was keen to do his duty. He had tackled her to the ground with a blow from his paw and was holding her down on the grass, his head a few centimetres from her nose, not making a sound. He wasn't even growling. You'd have thought he wanted to keep her there all day. The woman was terrified and didn't dare move for fear of being devoured. Given the size of the beast, good sense told me not to step in. I hurried off to fetch the animal's master. Blaise gave two or three instructions to his dog who immediately let his prey go. He seemed pretty pleased with himself, and so was I: another life saved!

GERVASUTTI PILLAR:
END IN SIGHT

● ● ● ● ● ● ● ● ●

My head was spinning. Five minutes of this gymkhana through séracs was enough and now I wanted to be sick! Paulo, the pilot of the Lama, had taken Giulio and me on board for the technical mission of the week. He headed into the maze that was the Bossons glacier, in the direction of the Grands Mulets. The clouds took it upon themselves to stop us from crossing the labyrinth of bridges and crevasses and Paulo swung us right then left, completely disorientating me, like being in a real-life 3D video game.

The Lama is the only solution for some rescues. It has the same Artouste engine as the Alouette III, but is 300 kilos lighter. The Alouette III's fittings are heavy and its cabin is larger, making it better adapted for carrying rescuers and injured climbers and walkers. Nevertheless, there is limited room for medical equipment once the stretcher has been taken on board. It is much better to have things prepared before you take off, as it is a bit cramped for any kind of procedure. The Lama doesn't have any of this paraphernalia and is noticeably more powerful than the Alouette. It holds the impressive altitude record of 11,000 metres and to set it the pilot, Jean Boulet, got rid of anything that wasn't absolutely necessary. He filled it up with aviation fuel and climbed up until the tank was empty, before letting it fall back down using auto-rotation.

Paulo didn't set the world altitude record but he must hold the record for the most hours flying in the massif. He has been around for the past twenty years and knows every nook and cranny. Flying with him reminds me of going on a roller-coaster ride as a kid. His skills at piloting his helicopter are near perfection. He has, nevertheless, been involved in four crashes and miraculously survived each one.

It only took us a few minutes to elude the traps on the Bossons glacier and reach the Cosmiques hut where there was acceptable visibility.

The PGHM had sent a team to the Rognon to try and locate the four Parisian castaways. A small group matching the description given had been spotted between two masses of cloud clinging to the Tacul. The Alouette had made two unsuccessful attempts but the wind was too strong. They couldn't pick them up, not even in a snatch and grab.

We had no idea what state our four climbers would be in and the atmospheric conditions were still bad. It is always a difficult call to make, as some people can put up with these conditions better than others with quite random consequences. There are many factors at play, including experience, equipment, fatigue and, most importantly, a person's emotional wherewithal.

Paulo had just gone over the 4,000-metre mark as we crossed the Col du Maudit. The helicopter was seized by yet more violent tremors but the cumulus clouds were starting to clear. The pilot took us around the pillar as our three pairs of eyes silently scrutinized the frieze of needle-sharp pinnacles.

Giulio and I had climbed what is a stunning route and we had a good idea where we might find them. And we were right. There were three figures on the saddle before the final section that takes you to the summit of the Tacul. This is a perfect spot to gather up makeshift bivouacs. They had got caught out right near the top.

'Right, let's winch them up while we can. We can't hang around and this isn't going to last,' said Paulo.

'Wait! Paulo, where's the fourth one?' asked Giulio, surprised.

'I can't see him. You'll have to take a look. I'll lower you down and carry on hovering.'

'Ok. Take us down.'

Paulo always appeared to be on a knife-edge: a mixture of unshakable skill and a permanent state of anxiety, a relentless strain.

Giulio shot down at high speed and then it was my turn. It was blowing from all directions and I could feel the violence of the shaking in the cable lowering me down. Giulio caught hold of my foot to pull me on to the ledge where the others were. The air was icy cold and it felt like we were in the middle of an austral winter. Here were three of the climbers we were looking for. They were frozen stiff and could barely answer our questions. They were covered in snow and ice and didn't seem to realize what was happening to them. Max's bulging eyes were in contrast with Olivier and Dod's lethargy.

'Hey, lads, you ok? We're from mountain rescue, we've come to collect you,' said Giulio.

'We'd given up hope,' Max finally managed to say.

'Can you stand up?'

'I don't know ...'

I examined them quickly. They were all conscious and Max couldn't stop shaking. He could barely get his words out. The two others were quieter. A little too quiet. They weren't trembling but I couldn't get any coherent answers to my questions. I was worried they had severe hypothermia, like the guys the week before. It looked like this year I would have all my hypothermia cases in the summer! Unfortunately, I couldn't get anything out of my broken tympanic thermometer. 'Fine bone china, handle them like fine bone china,' went Big Chief's voice, round and round in my head. Bone china or not, we had to get out of there quickly before we were stuck too. The spray of clouds was on the verge of closing up again and even if Giulio and I had enough gear to climb the route ourselves, we would never be able to take the others with us. Paulo was buzzing over our heads like a hornet, waiting for our signal. But where was the other climber?

We didn't have to look very far; we just had to follow the rope trapped behind a spike of rock. It was pulled tight and ten metres below an inert figure was hanging over the couloir of ice.

Rob had been delirious, seeing and hearing things the whole night long. He finally lost it and jumped.

We evacuated the living first and Paulo lowered them one at a time down to the Col du Midi where the Alouette III took over and flew them to hospital. We picked up Rob last, like a statue frozen for eternity. He would never marvel at anything and everything, like he used to do so well, ever again.

The cold had caused some damage. Two of the survivors had severe frostbite in their feet and the prognosis was pretty bleak. It was when I visited them later that I discovered the identity of their companion and it came as a complete shock. Rob had been a friend of mine and we had come through some memorable scrapes together but I hadn't seen him for ten years. I hadn't recognized his frost-ravaged features. He was the only one of the four not to have children and I couldn't help thinking that was why he didn't pull through.

Marianne called the hospital to find out how they were. She didn't leave a message.

PAWNS OF FATE

● ● ● ● ● ● ● ● ●

The white-skinned August holidaymakers had arrived, and their July counterparts had left, lobster red. Some days, without rhyme or reason, everything happened at once and there was pandemonium, others not.

'Nothing doing today? They don't want to fall, is that it? The weather's great, no storms in sight, the mountains are swarming with muppets and there's been nothing for us! Bugger!'

Matteo was irritated and the others had taken to calling him 'Crampon-that-pisses-me-off'. Originally from Italy's Aosta valley, he had dreamed about becoming a rescuer in Chamonix for five years. Now he had moved in with a petite and attractive Frenchwoman called Véronique and he wasn't in a hurry to leave. Today, though, he couldn't keep still and hadn't stopped whingeing.

'Something wrong, Matteo? Did we get out of the wrong side of bed this morning?' I teased him.

'I'm so bored! We've just been doing crappy little things today.'

'Don't worry. The storm will be here in an hour, everyone will go nuts and the phone'll ring off the hook.'

'Yeah, maybe. But that doesn't work for me. I don't fancy getting struck by lightning, storms aren't my thing. One day last year, when we were supposed to pick up some guys stuck on the top of the Charmoz, I thought I was never going to be able to grab the hook. It was full of static electricity. Jesus, it gave me such a shock! Dragon had to drag the hook over a rock to dissipate the charge. Storms really freak me out.'

It was true; we hadn't really done very much that day. Yet there were lots of people all over the mountains, so it was surprising we had had so few calls. We had come in that morning expecting to shatter all the records. In fact we had been on a small rescue flight earlier in the afternoon for a viper bite, which turned out not to be a viper bite. Having said that, you have to be careful with viper bites in August. I remember a tricky case I had when I was just starting out.

It was another beautiful but muggy day. I remember the weather, as that was the day we inaugurated the new fridge we had requested two years earlier. The air was clammy and humid and our clothes stuck to our skin.

René, an old pilot with the gendarmerie, was immersed in a chess match with Henri, which looked like it would go on for some time. Neither one could get the other into mate and they were doggedly battling it out to the death, taking each other's pieces one by one.

Outside people were reading or chatting. There were even two men playing pétanque behind the small chalet we used as an office before the present DZ building became operational.

The day had started at first light with a reconnaissance flight. We were looking for a couple of climbers who had set out to do the traverse of the Grandes Jorasses and there had been no word since. They had in fact turned around, returning safely without telling anyone.

Following this, apart from two exhausted climbers on Mont Blanc and a gastroenteritis victim at the Couvercle hut, our activity subsided as the heat grew in intensity.

The telephone rang for a long time before anyone answered it. Finally, Henri gave in and picked up the receiver.

'Hello, is that the DZ?'

'Yeah.'

'We've had a call. You've got to get moving.'

'What is it?'

'Someone's been bitten by a viper in Samoëns, Fer-à-Cheval.'

'Got any more info?'

'It's on the chalets du Boret path at the World's End.'

'Weeell, I'm not sure we'll be able to tear René away from his game of chess …'

'Stop mucking around, according to the caller the guy's not well. You'd better take the doc. The bloke's wearing a yellow T-shirt and is with a woman. The third member of the group went for help.'

'Right, we're on our way.'

And we were off again.

By this time, viper bites were already quite trivial affairs. Yet when I was in the Scouts the description was very different. It was an emergency case, the venom had to be sucked out, you had to use a tourniquet – the whole works! I imagined myself making an incision in the wound with a penknife to remove the venom. In fact, in my time as a doctor I had never seen anyone not survive a viper bite. But then, experts in the field could never agree among themselves on a treatment strategy: should you give heparin, steroids, start serotherapy, do nothing? How do you decide? Despite all the progress made in medical science, we didn't really know what to suggest to the panicked patients who turned up at A&E, having been bitten. Besides, most of the time they haven't been bitten by a snake at all, and have been stung by a wasp or pricked themselves on a thistle. And when it really is a viper bite, it often happens that it bites but doesn't inject any venom.

It took ages to find the man and you'd have thought he had never learned about distress signals. The helicopter finally dropped us off near a man lying on the ground. He was pale and looked upset. A ninety-kilo baby.

'Hello, sir, I'm an emergency doctor. How are you feeling?'

Nothing.

'Sir? Are you ok?'

'No, an animal's bitten me!'

'What kind of animal? A snake?'

'No, it was … It looked like a big blue lizard. With teeth … I didn't get a good look at it.'

He looked like a proper mummy's boy: barely weaned and a bit of a wimp. I didn't really believe his snake bite story. He showed me a red patch on his hand that looked nothing like fang marks and his general state gave me no cause for alarm. His blood pressure was fine. And his pulse was a bit fast, but that's normal for someone in an emotional state who has just seen a huge helicopter land five metres from him for the first time in his life. I tried to reassure him but it was in vain, as he was convinced he had been bitten by a monster. I invited him to climb aboard the helicopter and go with us to Chamonix hospital and he duly accepted.

The flight should have been a quiet affair. The spectacle of all the little hikers lifting up their heads to watch the helicopter made me chuckle. Then when we were halfway there, the trip took a turn for the worse. My patient suddenly went pale and limp. His pulse had become thready, just like the descriptions of viper bite cases in medical textbooks. Was there something to his snake story? To set my mind at rest, I injected him in the buttock with 120 milligrams of methylprednisolone, a corticosteroid that prevents the patient from going into anaphylactic shock. Given his weight, he needed at least that. It didn't look like he was getting any better and we took him straight to the hospital without stopping at the DZ first.

When I went back to see him in hospital a couple of hours later, the intensive care unit was getting a good scrubbing. The lino was being mopped and a rather unpleasant *Toilet Duck* kind of smell assailed my nostrils.

My patient was half-comatose, clammy and white as a sheet. My colleague at A&E didn't think he looked great when I had handed him over. He also hadn't really bought the snake bite theory. Yet, given that the patient was turning grey, he thought it prudent to keep him in the intensive care unit for observation.

A few minutes earlier, Big Chief had visited the patient with a nurse, and it was his turn to peer over the strange case. He too had his doubts about the cause of the man's eclectic collection of symptoms. The nurse, who was none other than Cécile, my future wife, and Big Chief stopped at the bottom of his bed, the former awaiting orders from the latter, the other rubbing his chin looking for clues.

During this time the patient was lying there quietly, perhaps too quietly. All that could be heard was the whistle of the oxygen he was being given through a mask.

Big Chief looked distractedly out of the window, in front of which passed a paraglider who had missed the official landing field at the Clos du Savoie. 'Another client for us,' Big Chief was heard to say.

Suddenly, their attention was caught by the grimace on the patient's face. He had turned from an off-white colour to blue, his muscles had tensed and he started to writhe around. His face now went crimson and his body was shaking as if he was about to go into convulsions. Neither Big Chief nor the nurse knew what to do.

'Is everything ok, sir? Are you in pain?' tried Cécile.

It was impossible to get anything out of him.

'It looks like he has stomach ache,' came Big Chief's comment.

'Give him a vial of Spasfon to start off, with eighty milligrams of Solumedrol. Let's see if that calms him down. What did we give him just now?'

'Five hundred of Ringer and 500 of Plasmion. But his pressure's between 9 and 10,' replied Cécile.

'I don't understand what's happening. Whatever it is, it doesn't look like a snake bite!'

'Could it be a wasp sting or something like that, doctor?'

'Well, maybe …'

Big Chief was rubbing his chin again, still sceptical. Cécile gave the patient the injection but it didn't calm him down at all. It looked like he was trying to say something but nothing would come. He was bright red and still moaning. A couple of minutes went by when, all of a sudden, a few words escaped his lips. It almost sounded like a sentence and Big Chief and Cécile rushed towards him, trying to get him to say it again. But once again the sentence remained inaudible and they leaned in closer.

Fatal mistake! There was an explosion. It was like the return of *The Exorcist*! A jet of vomit was sprayed two metres into the air. In a single movement, Big Chief and Cécile desperately jumped backwards out of the way. But it was too late; two further fountains of sick, almost as powerful as the first one, flooded the room. Big Chief had got it all over his shirt. He wasn't happy and was cursing. The room was filled with a foetid odour from the bowels of Hell itself... The patient's sphincters had given way too, and he was leaking from all his orifices. Big Chief and Cécile contemplated the damage, feeling sick, their arms hanging limply at their sides.

'Oh poo! I've got it all over my top!' exclaimed Cécile who makes a point of never swearing in front of patients.

Big Chief looked despondently at her, declaring, 'I don't like this job ...'

We never did find out what kind of beast it was that had bitten him.

It was three in the afternoon and, as I had predicted, the storm broke over Mont Blanc and the telephone started ringing. Matteo sprang up to answer.

'A rescue request at the Requin. A guy's peeled off the Renaudi. The hut guardian can see him. It looks like he's hanging on one of the middle pitches,' announced Matteo with an almost triumphant tone.

'What's the weather like at the hut? It doesn't look good from here,' asked Jules, the pilot, with concern, looking up at the Mer de Glace.

'He said it was looking ok for the time being but we'll have to be quick.'

The DZ was a hive of activity. Everyone had a job to do, what with the winch, the drill and the static rope.

Two journalists had been waiting for the opportunity to get some rescue footage for the TF1 eight o'clock news bulletin for two days. But they were out of luck this time, as at that precise moment their cameraman was getting sandwiches at the local café. The two Parisians tried to work out what was going on but the rescue team members were too busy sorting out the gear to waste time on explanations. We were going to leave them on the bench for the most interesting rescue of the day, as they would be in the way. To cap it all, the cameraman, who was supposed to fly with us and take the pictures, was also the chubbiest of the three of them. He was wearing big, completely impractical, plastic boots and a hunter's jacket covered in pockets that were full of lenses and extra batteries. It hung loosely over his belly, catching on everything.

For my part, I was ready. I took two seconds to lace up the boots that I can't wear for more than ten minutes when I'm in the valley. We ushered the two or three kids, who had come to see their daddies saving lives, into the office where they wouldn't get sliced into little pieces and took off at breakneck speed.

The Renaudi on the Dent du Requin is a classic route. The team in distress wasn't difficult to spot. One of the climbers, who must have been the second, was pressed up against the belay stance above, while the other climber, the one who had taken the fall, was dangling in space below. Jules was hovering over the scene so that we could assess the situation. Matteo, who was leading the rescue party, gave out instructions.

'Ok, Jules, drop Manu at the Requin hut while we consolidate the stance. I'll call you.'

'Will you need back up?' asked Jules.

'Not yet, it should be ok.'

Jules dropped me off at the hut's landing pad. The guardian was waiting to fill me in. He started explaining things before the helicopter even left and I didn't catch much of what he was saying.

'There's a guy and a girl. They set off this morning. I heard shouting and I went out to have a look. The guy was dangling there like a sausage and it didn't take long to figure out what had happened.'

This didn't tell me that much more, apart from the fact that one of them was a woman and she wasn't the one who was hurt. I turned on my radio to hear how Matteo and Nanard were getting on being winched down the fateful pitch.

Nanard quickly put me in the picture.

'The guy's pretty banged up ... He's bleeding around his pelvis and he's in a lot of pain. I'll bring you up.'

'Ok. I'm ready.'

'Watch out, we're hanging in space.'

The helicopter was already above me and with the noise I couldn't make out Nanard's last sentence. Fred, the mechanic opened the door for me and I dived into the machine's belly. I didn't have time to put my cabin helmet back on to hear where they were going to dump me. But I didn't think it was going to be somewhere nice. The door opened again. I was sitting at the back with my bag between my legs. Fred handed me the hook and I clipped it into the large screw-link on my harness.

'Ready to be kicked out?'

I gave him a thumbs up. I was hauled upwards violently, and thankfully I had a helmet on by this point. The door opened over nothingness. I was jettisoned into the void on the end of a five millimetre cable. Everything was spinning, the wind, the rock, the gusts of air …

Nanard caught me by the hand. I had all the gear clipped to me: the twenty-kilo stretcher, the KED to immobilize head, neck and spine, my backpack, I was like a proper Christmas tree. The slab was as smooth as a baby's bottom and I couldn't find the slightest hold for my feet. Stowing gear was going to be complicated! We couldn't afford to drop a single piece of equipment. Matteo was above us, with the victim's girlfriend. He had added a couple of friends to back up the belay and had set up a static rope to which we could attach the stretcher. Nanard clipped me in, I unhooked from the winching cable and the helicopter flew off with the female climber.

We were alone with a job to do. Nanard explained what we had:

'He's called Bernard and there's blood pissing out of his left buttock. I don't want to touch him!'

Our patient Bernard was moaning but we could see that he was tough and was doing his best to control himself, trying not to complain. His face was ashen and contorted in pain. Great beads of blood were coming through his beige canvas trousers, forming a huge dark patch. Not a good sign. I had to try and think straight and not drop anything. This time the medical side was all important, not just to ease the pain but also to stop the patient from possibly bleeding to death.

It was his pelvis. I had to be organized but I also had to act quickly. We sometimes rush things when there's actually no need to hurry. Yet in this situation we had to act quickly as the stance was particularly uncomfortable, the weather was threatening to come in and blood was pouring out of the victim.

Nanard saw me hesitate and guessed what I was thinking.

'Manu, think we'd better evacuate him straight away and take him to the hut? We don't want to get stuck here!'

'Hang on while I see how he is …'

Bernard was hanging from the rope attached to his harness and Nanard had also clipped him into a bolt that happened to be there.

I felt his torso and pelvis to get an idea of the damage. It didn't look like he had hit his head, and that was something at least! Feeling his bones move and crack under my fingers, confirmed a diagnosis of an open fracture of the iliac crest. Bugger. It was impossible to tell if the compression exerted by the harness was limiting the haemorrhaging or was exacerbating his state by reducing the venous return. I could feel him slipping away. I couldn't get a radial pulse and his blood pressure was in his boots. I had to make a decision straight away, without letting my voice betray my hesitation.

'We'll finish him off if we take him like this now. I have to get some fluids into him.'

'Are you sure?' asked Nanard.

'Yeah, just give me five minutes.'

I was far from sure but the conviction with which I gave my reply helped me convince myself it was the right thing to do. It had been a long time since anyone had questioned one of my decisions, at least openly. The rescuers I worked with now were all younger than me. I had more than fifteen years of rescues to my name and I sensed that they trusted me.

I was reminded of other rescues, memories of my first intubations. I remembered the fateful day when we had been called to a piste at the Grands Montets for a head injury.

It was the middle of the ski season but it hadn't snowed for over three weeks. The piste, as hard as a bowling alley with rocks sticking out here and there, was nevertheless full of people. A young woman had fallen over 150 metres down a slope, probably hitting two or three rocks as she went, and had a head like a football.

I had little experience in intubations and dreaded actually having to do them. The woman's eye sockets were so swollen that I couldn't even open her eyes to check the dilation of her pupils. She was agitated and was twisting around and moaning, not knowing where or who she was. A few years earlier, a patient like this wouldn't have received any kind of pre-hospital medical care as there wasn't a doctor attached to the rescue service. The victim would have been forcibly strapped to the stretcher and whisked off to hospital. Having a doctor there was a good thing, as long as they were actually capable of administering emergency care. In the case of serious head trauma, we had been pumped full of recommended courses of action. The most important and urgent of these was to sedate the patient completely to ensure adequate oxygen supply to the brain with assisted ventilation. There is a risk of irreversible brain damage if it is deprived of oxygen for more than three minutes.

The atmosphere was tense and members of the skier's family were panicking. Ski patrollers were doing their best to hold the woman still and two or three holidaymakers, claiming to be in the medical profession, offered their help. One was a cardiologist, another was a hospital porter. And I was expected to stay cool, calm and collected with all those pairs of eyes watching my every move! I had the crucial decision to make: did I put her to sleep and intubate her? Which meant, doing it properly. Or did I chicken out, tie her up the old-fashioned way and get her to hospital and into the care of my more hard-boiled colleagues as quickly as possible? I went for the braver option, to actually do my job.

And it went very badly. Firstly, the patient managed to rip out her drip twice and just as I was about to inject her with the sedative, Etomidate, I lost the syringe in the snow. My bag was in a complete mess as people had trodden on it. Idiots! As, at that time, I couldn't use a curare, it took me three tries to get the tube in the right hole. I was taking so long that one of the rescue team asked me sarcastically if I wanted to cut my losses and have her taken to hospital as she was. I was sweating buckets.

Once in the helicopter I realized I had taken so long that the oxygen bottle was empty and I had to ventilate my patient with a bag valve mask as she was starting to come round.

That was fifteen years ago but it felt very recent …

'Manu, want me to take your bag?' suggested Nanard.

'No, it's fine. I can use it to work on.'

Once again I would be able to make good use of it. I had clipped it to the left of Bernard and was using it as a tray. I had managed, with relative ease, to get an IV-line into the patient, hooked up to a saline pouch.

'Hurry up, Manu! The clouds are coming in. Dragon won't be able to pick us up,' came Matteo's worried commentary from thirty metres above our heads.

'It's ok. I'll get the fentanyl into him and we can put him in the stretcher.'

Up until then everything had been going more or less ok. We decided not to use the stretcher and to put him in the KED instead. That way his arms and legs were free and we could winch him up using the brace and not his harness, trying not to dislodge his pelvis. The problem now was sorting out the ropes, identifying the ones we could cut away and those that had to stay. The patient's blood pressure looked stable and the saline IV had probably given him a boost. But the steady trickle of blood wasn't slowing down and it was impossible to assess where it was coming from, now that his trousers were drenched in it.

'Fuck. It's clouding over!' shouted Matteo.

'Come in, Dragon,' said Nanard.

'This is Dragon. Go ahead.'

'We're ready for winching, but it's clouding over, I don't know if you can get through,' explained Nanard.

'Tell him to do his best. It's really touch and go here!' I insisted.

'We're coming. We'll see what we can do,' came the reply.

Bernard was out of it. The powerful analgesic I had given him had knocked him out but his breathing was ok. He looked very grey and I wondered what was going through his mind at that moment. Maybe his life was passing in front of his eyes?

The fentanyl had probably got rid of the pain and he had completely surrendered. He wasn't showing any more signs of struggle.

This makes our job a whole lot easier. The simple fact that the patients weren't feeling any pain any more gave us the sense of having got the job half done already. Yet we can never afford to stop at that and in cases such as this one it was still an emergency. Cardiac arrest during the winching stage is the most dreaded complication. As the patient wasn't in the stretcher he was going to have to be upright during the manoeuvre. The pooling of blood in the flaccid lower limbs can lead to fatal cardiac arrest. We would have avoided this problem if we had been able to winch the patient up flat in the stretcher.

Dragon was flying around trying to get to us, and we could hear it going left and then coming back right. There was a rumble of thunder in the distance. The storm was near and it scared us half to death. Suddenly, after several dozen interminable minutes of waiting, Dragon appeared above us. We heard Fred say to us, 'Hand him over pronto. It's pretty dicey out here. We can't stay long!'

The hook had already been lowered down. I saw Nanard hesitate for a fraction of a second before cutting the rope. Thankfully, he got the right one.

Bernard flew off into the clouds, spinning as he went, which can't have helped his state of shock. Then we saw nothing more, the clouds had closed up again. Nanard looked at me, relieved.

'Well, he got away ok!'

'Let's hope he makes it to hospital ...'

I was far from relieved. For the rescuers retrieving the victim was where their job ended, but for the doctors that was where it started. I was worried about the extent of his injuries and it depended on exactly what they were. A fractured pelvis can bleed so much that a surgeon can really struggle just to stop the blood loss. They sometimes have to rush the patient to a teaching hospital. If the pelvis has been shattered into several pieces, the only way to stop the bleeding is to embolise the ruptured arteries before the damaged area. This technique is only carried out in large specialist centres.

'Dragon to Crampons,' we heard over the radio.

'We're listening,' replied Nanard.

'It's gonna be tricky picking up the doc. The clouds have come in again ...'

'Take him straight to the DZ at the hospital and tell them to get the resuss room ready!' I instructed.

'Ok. Roger that!'

The humming of the helicopter got fainter, leaving us in the cotton wool-like silence of the mist that enveloped us like a spider in its web.

We couldn't just hang around waiting for it to warm up again. It was entirely possible that Dragon wouldn't be able to get back to us. The euphoria we had felt at the relative ease with which we had rescued our man gave way to a slightly deflated feeling that wasn't made any better by the bitter cold. We were feeling the cold all the more for our T-shirts being covered in sweat. We hadn't thought about this as we were leaping into action. Now that the pressure was off, a shudder went through me. The message was clear: we were on our own and had to get out of this by ourselves. There were four pitches to get down with all the gear and the wet snow, which had started to fall, was not going to make it easy. And we also had the stretcher, which couldn't be taken up with the patient as he was in the KED brace. Perfect.

It took us a good hour to get to the bottom of the face. The snow at the bergschrund was rotten and we fell up to our knees into a sorbet of coarse salt-like crystals.

Matteo declared authoritatively, 'We're not going to piss around taking all this gear back to the hut. It'll be better if we stash all this stuff here somewhere and come back and get it tomorrow when the weather's cleared.'

Nanard and I were wholly in favour of this idea. Matteo's choice of hiding place for the equipment, however, did surprise us. I don't know why, but he decided to drag the stretcher to a small overhang next to a narrow couloir full of snow and rubble.

To reach it, he had to cross a small patch of névé snow just above the gaping bergschrund. It didn't look like a particularly safe place to me and Nanard didn't think so either. He didn't mind telling Matteo.

'Be careful, that doesn't look good. It's really unstable underneath.'

We dumbly let him get on with it, staying where we were. As he was pulling the stretcher, the patch of snow detached itself from the slope and came away above him. His shoes slid and the crampons might have been of use after all, if he had bothered to put them back on. At first he didn't want to let go of the stretcher, which was sliding towards the crevasse. Then, when he realized he couldn't get a grip on the rotten snow, he let go but it was too late. The entire patch of snow above gave way, knocking him off his feet. He flailed around wildly but couldn't find anything to hold on to. Then he disappeared into the bergschrund. We had been powerless to help. In the fraction of a second before he vanished his eyes met mine, as if he wanted to say something. No doubt it was 'Say goodbye to Véro for me ...'

Nanard threw himself on his pack, looking for the shovel he had just put away, while I stayed rooted to the spot. A second snow slide came down, not looking like it was going to stop any time soon, and filled up the crevasse that had just swallowed up Matteo. This wasn't happening to me, it had to be a nightmare. How could such an ordinary situation turn into a tragedy so quickly?

Before he even knew what was happening to him, Matteo had been buried under four metres of snow. It was atrocious.

Nanard ran to the top of the crevasse, which was completely choked with snow, and started to dig as fast as he could. I joined him and tried to clear away the snow as best I could with my hands and arms. But the inescapable truth was overwhelming: there were at least two tonnes of waterlogged snow in the crevasse. The helicopter couldn't get in to bring reinforcements and we only had our hands and one miserable shovel.

We stopped two hours later, utterly exhausted, not daring to look at each other and filled with a strange feeling of guilt. I was freezing cold even though I was drenched in sweat.

A little earlier, Nanard had managed to summon up the wherewithal to call Cordial. After a few exchanges, panic spread among the rescuers at the DZ. We had heard the helicopter flying round and round above the clouds, trying to get through the misty ceiling separating us from the valley. On board were the avalanche dog and our friends. Dragon finally managed to drop them off at the Requin hut. Yet, in any case, it was always going to be too late by the time they got to us.

Matteo's arm finally appeared. I was under no illusions as to his fate. I knew the reality of the situation far too well: survival is rare indeed after the victim has been buried for forty-five minutes, unless there is an air pocket around their mouth. And even if that is the case, the victim will end up being poisoned by the carbon dioxide he or she has exhaled. We were dreaming if we thought he could survive for two hours under the dense and heavy pack of snow. Matteo was blue and lifeless. I got out the resuscitation kit without conviction. I couldn't *not* try to do something, even though I knew it was hopeless. My hands were completely frozen and I was utterly exhausted and good sense should have told me to stop. I put the oxygen mask on the wrong way round and forced the tube into him. I couldn't get over the fact that I was doing this to a friend. I knew very well that it was over and this knowledge coloured everything I did.

The rescue team finally arrived, the dog first, excited at the prospect of work. Completely overwhelmed, Blaise distractedly tried to calm him down. There was nothing else that could be done. We stood there, useless and shivering in the cold next to his lifeless body. Nanard got a survival blanket out of his bag. In spite of myself I found that I was thinking how inappropriate the term 'survival' was now. We rolled Matteo up in it to take him to a more stable spot. The helicopter would pick him up when the weather improved.

My gear was strewn all over the ground, draining into the snow. I felt like dumping it all in the crevasse. We couldn't work miracles and the extent of our limitations seemed brutally stark to me. All those years of studying and training, all the energy I had put into it for so long, all for this. I was nothing, a pawn that fate could sweep away with the back of its hand when the time came. Matteo's time had come: he was gone.

Before we covered up his body, Jeannot, one of the old guard, in a final act of frustrated anger, gave him a whack as if chastising him for getting himself caught. Undoubtedly Matteo wasn't the first of his friends he'd seen go.

To make matters worse, there were a string of serious accidents that week and Mont Blanc was in the headlines for a large part of August.

It hadn't snowed at altitude for over ten days and the final section of ridge on the normal route up Mont Blanc was as smooth and glassy as marble. Day after day novice climbers were being caught out on the descent and we picked up three teams in pieces. There were even calls from certain quarters to block access to the route, the press stirring up the furore.

I thought we should start by banning the use of ropes. Ropes are for holding people, not dragging partners down too, as the old prints showed only too well. The descent from Mont Blanc's summit via the Bosses Ridge is not difficult when there is a good track in compact snow, but there are huge drops on either side. Now everyone knows that most of the climbers taking the normal route are beginners, a minority of whom can afford to take a guide. The benefit of having a guide is that he or she is expected to know how to short rope a client down an ice slope. The technique involves holding up the client even before he or she has fallen, the rope being held tight every step of the way, and that's the bit people don't understand. It only takes the person at the back, supposed to be holding the one at the front, to look away for a second as the other catches his or her crampon in a baggy bit of gaiter for an accident to happen. Fifty centimetres of slack in the rope is enough to cause what is known in the jargon as the cork effect. The shock on the rope is strong enough to pull everyone off their feet.

And there are certain places where you simply cannot afford to fall.

FEELING THE HEAT

• • • • • • • • •

'Hurry up, Gaston! At this rate we'll miss the Plan de l'Aiguille lift.'

'My feet are rubbed raw. These new shoes were a bloody stupid idea. I should have used my old leather boots. And I'm boiling. I can't take much more of this!'

'Why don't you take your down jacket off? You're gonna explode if we carry on at this rate.'

'There isn't enough room in my bag. I'd have to take everything out and put it back in again. We haven't got time.'

Alain had just about had enough. He'd really hit the jackpot with this client. He seemed like a nice enough chap at the start. He was in his fifties with the slight paunch of a man who wanted to get fit and prove he could climb Mont Blanc. He said he had started training again, doing two five-kilometre runs a week and cutting down on the cigarettes. But that morning he couldn't stop wheezing.

When Alain had been to visit him a couple of days before, he had put away a handsome amount of hooch. Gaston had drunk three glasses of the stuff down in one before Alain had even finished his first. In short, he liked his food and drink a bit too much but was highly motivated.

Gaston had talked incessantly for the entire afternoon the day before. It had given Alain a migraine and the only thing that helped him when he had a migraine was complete silence. But his client gabbled on, spouting one inanity after another about those foolhardy people who didn't employ guides and then called out the rescue service at the drop of a hat.

Gaston was really feeling the effects of the altitude as they set off down the ridge starting at the top station of the Aiguille du Midi cable car. His heart was beating ten to the dozen and he made gaffe after gaffe, the kind of thing that really winds a guide up. First he dropped a glove, then there were the rental crampons that were supposed to be set up for his boots, but which needed adjusting with a Leather-man. He was impetuous and uncoordinated, the kind of person with whom you could expect pretty much anything to happen. And although Alain had taken him on a training route the year before they had to start everything from scratch. He trod on the rope with his crampons on the descent but Alain had kept his cool and bitten his tongue. The best thing to do with people like this was to stay calm and not get them any more agitated!

Each safe step on the descent of the ridge was a small miracle as Gaston nearly fell at least three times. After having lifted his eyes to heaven in exasperation, Alain decided to keep them riveted to his companion's heels to anticipate the next blunder.

The evening in the Cosmiques hut brought Gaston back to the realities of the environment and the joys of limited oxygen at altitude. The bottle of red he ordered, against Alain's advice, really knocked him out and before he knew where he was he was having difficulty getting his words out and had to go to bed early like an overgrown kid.

He was far from radiant when they got up later that night to set off. He was drawn with bags under his eyes. He had been plagued by the strangest nightmares all night and his dearest wish was to be left to vomit quietly on his own. The weather wasn't looking very good either: fog high up with a few clouds, bright spells in the afternoon and a forecast reliability of three out of five. In the meantime, it was snowing.

After half an hour of indecisiveness on Gaston's part, Alain managed to persuade him to at least try to climb Mont Blanc du Tacul. Gaston was resigned to it and after taking a couple of aspirins was feeling better. The weather was completely over-cast and Alain wasn't sure they would get very far on their climb. Half the Mont Blanc climbers had gone back to bed and there was no mad scramble of teams to get to the track.

Gaston perked up and got his second wind. The weather hadn't worsened by the time they got to the shoulder on the Tacul. It had even stopped snowing. They could make out a few bright patches in the dim light of the early morning. Gaston said he felt strong enough to have a go at the steep slope on the Mont Maudit. The climb required much more effort and he started to feel the altitude again. Not without a little difficulty, they finally reached the col at nine-fifteen. Gaston was shat-tered but spurred on by the good weather that was coming in slowly but surely. He wanted to go on.

The walk up to the summit felt like it would never end. After the Col de la Brenva their already modest pace slowed further still. Yet Gaston carried on. There was virtually no wind and the sun was beating down on them. That was when Gaston realized he had left his sunglasses on the table in the hut. What next? thought Alain, as he lent Gaston his own pair. The summit didn't seem to be getting any closer. They finally reached it at one in the afternoon. Gaston was utterly exhausted but the weather was holding and it was very hot.

The descent was epic. Gaston could barely stay on his feet, his natural clumsiness exacerbated by fatigue. Alain had to be extra vigilant.

The sun was blisteringly hot.

The walk down the Petit Plateau was excruciating. Gaston was sweating buckets and collapsed every fifty metres. Alain only had one thing on his mind: get to the shelter of Plan de l'Aiguille lift where he could shade his eyes. He felt a complete idiot for having forgotten his spare pair of glasses. He could feel his eyes were burning, aggravated by beads of sweat.

Three hours later, as they were making their way up towards the old Glaciers lift station, Alain sensed a burst of energy in Gaston. He had stopped speaking and was breathing hard, powering ahead like an ox, his shoulders hunched forward.

'Slow down, Gaston. You can't keep this pace up all the way to the Plan station.'

No reply.

'Gaston! You hear me? Slow down!'

'Yeah …'

But Gaston wasn't slowing down at all. They had taken off the rope once they left the glacier and Alain had let him go in front. He ran after him. Gaston seemed to be in his own little world, on a military-style route march. This was unsettling in a man who was usually so chatty and extrovert.

Alain was starting to worry. He had never had to deal with this kind of situation before.

At a bend in the moraine, Gaston took the left-hand path leading down to the valley instead of the right-hand one that would take them to the lift station.

'Right, Gaston. Go right! What are you doing?' shouted Alain.

'I'll do it. You'll see. I'll do it,' replied Gaston.

But it was no longer the same man speaking, he sounded like an automaton.

Alain ran up to him, grabbing him by the sleeve.

'You ok, Gaston? What's the matter with you?'

'Gotta keep going … Keep going …'

Gaston was delirious. He was bright red and stared at Alain, half-crazed. He's lost it, thought Alain. He tried to pull him in, to get him to sit down on a boulder. The blow came out of the blue. Alain ducked instinctively, only half dodging the ice axe that Gaston seemed intent on driving into his skull. His forehead was bleeding but that was the least of his worries! My God, this is a dangerous job! thought Alain, dumbfounded. Gaston wrenched himself free and ran off through the boulders.

Taken aback, Alain watched him zigzag down the slope as if he was under machine-gun fire, clinging to everything as he went. Before long the inevitable happened: as he went behind a scree slope his feet caught in some rocks and he fell head first. Lucky he's still wearing his helmet, thought Alain as he ran after him. As he got to him Gaston tried to stand up and Alain grabbed him by the torn collar of his down jacket.

'For Christ's sake, Gaston, stop! What's the matter with you? Hey, Gaston! Answer me!'

'Shut your face!... Come on! We've got to keep going. Shit, your ice axe! Use your bloody ice axe!'

'Calm down, Gaston. It's me, Alain.'

'Come on! Look out, stop doing that ... I told you to use your ice axe!'

Gaston had completely lost it. It looked like he was reliving the route in some kind of waking nightmare. He stared at Alain with his sun-reddened panic-stricken eyes before maniacally setting off again.

'Mountain rescue. Come in, mountain rescue, this is a mountain guide. Mountain rescue? Can you hear me?'

It was the late afternoon. At the DZ Raoul was taking his nephew's radio cassette player apart at the table upstairs in the common room. He stopped what he was doing to listen to the call. Apparently Cordial wasn't answering, unless the gendarme on duty was away from his desk for a few seconds. He reluctantly put down the small tools he had in his hands and answered the call using the base microphone.

'This is mountain rescue. Who's this calling?'

'It's Alain Chardon, I'm a guide. I've got a serious problem: my client's done a runner!'

He sounded like he had just been in a fight and was trying to get his breath back.

'You've lost your client?' said Raoul with surprise.

'No, I know where he is and I'm running after him. He's gone completely nuts!'

Raoul was bemused and looked at the microphone as if it might be a joke. But his practical side and sense of professionalism told him to stick to the standard questions.

'What is your position?'

'Below the Glaciers station. He's heading downhill. I've got to catch him!'

'Ok. We're coming in the helicopter.'

That morning I was pretty relaxed when I got to the DZ. It was forecast to be cloudy in the afternoon but nothing to worry about. The weather wasn't too bad although it was a bit muggy. I had set about tidying the piles of stuff we didn't use in the medical storeroom.

I sometimes wonder if I'm becoming too much of a nag as I can't bear to work in a mess. Coffee cup rings on the floor, snowboard magazines all over the place, stinking rubbish bags, forgotten gloves and dubious-looking old socks; I can't tolerate any of it any more.

One likes to think that anything to do with the medical profession has to be spick and span, even sterilized, and that doctors must be real sticklers for keeping things clean and tidy. Around here it is the gendarmes who are always in their Sunday best: never a hair out of place, their vehicles spotless and equipment tidied away. The Chamonix doctors, on the other hand, are anything but domestic goddesses and the medical store was a complete mess.

I tidy things when it doesn't look like we will be called out. One of my colleagues says I must have some kind of OCD (Obsessive-Compulsive Disorder) that comes out when I'm feeling down. I closed the door and started with a massacre of the flies. My record is forty-five flies in less than fifteen minutes. My technique never fails and consists in swatting the fly where it takes off and not where it is. I don't miss many.

Once I've let off steam and the sweeping is done, I throw myself into my writing. I specialize in articles on frostbite. It is a bit of a niche market as Chamonix is one of the rare places in the world where one can treat victims with fresh frostbite injuries, that is just after they have got off the mountain. There are few teams working on it elsewhere as they don't have the patients. It is not difficult to become a specialist in this area and there isn't much competition. I am invited all over the world and, for the time being, I don't mind at all. All the more so because I am often invited to mountainous regions where I can make the most of my trip and go climbing.

I can't resist a single publication, be it in French, English or Spanish. It often feels like I am repeating myself when I am writing my articles but it keeps my little grey cells active. I spend a lot of time constructing and changing my sentences to convey a maximum amount of information in a minimum amount of space. It is the opposite of writing a novel. The work is a bit like a drug as it is often quite late by the time I finish writing.

'Oi, you ready, doc? There's a guy gone mad under the old Glaciers cable car station and his guide's running after him,' explained Raoul, adjusting his helmet.

'A guy gone mad? Just what I've always thought: you have to be mad to do this sport! What's the matter with him?'

'Dunno, we're going to have a look. You'd better take a shot of something for him!'

As if I was in the habit of turning up empty-handed! I must confess, I didn't really feel like going and was focused on something else. I had finished tidying up and was making the most of the lull to sort out a few extremely important equipment issues. I had taken my trumpet apart to grease the valves and my video camera gear was spread out on the desk, as I wanted to sort it out. It was all over the place and all of it was precious. Neither was I in my 'speedy departure' clothes, as the firemen call it. My Bermuda shorts, T-shirt and sandals meant I was in more of a 'beach departure' mode. It was always the same, you only had to relax for a second and the radio would start spluttering into life again. There was nothing I could do, I was just going to have to get changed.

'Watch out for the cables, Jean-Jacques.'

'Yeah, I can see them.'

'Paraglider at eleven o'clock.'

'Ok.'

'Another one at twelve o'clock.'

'Seen it.'

This was the usual conversation between the pilot and mechanic and it quickly got us in rescue mode. Raoul looked to the right and I looked left. I scrutinized the ground shortsightedly, looking for a nutcase gallivanting through the scrubby mountainside. He wasn't easy to spot in the rocky terrain, especially as he had had the bright idea of wearing green.

'I see him,' shouted Raoul.

'Where?' asked Jean-Jacques.

'There, under us. You've just passed him. Go around again.'

He wasn't galloping any more. The guide had caught him and motioned to us with one hand while with the other trying to hold down his client, who was struggling like a man possessed.

'Ok. I'll winch you down. Get ready, Raoul.'

Raoul adjusted his harness, unplugged his microphone from the cabin system and checked the fat karabiner on his harness, into which Fred had clipped the cable. The doors opened and he was lowered down.

The mechanic's description of what was happening meant the pilot knew exact what was going on without having to take his eyes off the fir tree right in front of him.

Now it was my turn to be lowered, whirling around, down into the warmth of the larches.

'Calm down, Gaston! Everything's going to be fine.'

I immediately recognized the guide, not by his badge but because I bumped into him quite regularly. He was quietly spoken and careful. I had helped him out two or three times when he had had migraines. He would get them at altitude, which was kind of a drag for a guide. He always greeted me by my first name and I regularly forgot his. As with everyone else who spends too much time at high altitudes, I am starting to suffer from short-term memory loss. I can remember faces but not names.

The guide was holding his client down as best he could. He gave me a strained look and I saw the blood trickling down his head. I still had no idea it was his client who had whacked him with his ice axe! The guide was dripping with sweat and was sitting astride his client, pinning him to the ground, and was obviously very pleased to see us. The guy underneath looked completely mad. With the whites of his eyes showing, he looked like he was ready to kill someone.

Raoul hesitated for a second before putting out his hand to the guide. Which of them was the nutter? The din of the helicopter above, the crackling radio and the bellowing from the client gave the whole scene a slightly surreal feel. Where was I again? The guide's shouts brought me back to reality.

'Help me! I can't hold him any longer. He's nuts!'

The man being held down was squealing like a pig, his roars drowning out our conversation. Raoul finally decided to act. He tried to hold Gaston down. One of them did look more cracked than the other after all. The helicopter pilot finally realized he was in the way and flew off. We could speak at last.

Alain explained as best he could.

'He just lost it and ran off down the mountainside. I had to run after him and tackle him!'

'What's his name?' asked Raoul.

'Gaston. And I'm Alain. He's my client.'

Gaston was wriggling around all over the place. He wasn't having any of it.

'Right, doc, what do we do?' said Raoul impatiently.

'Well, there's not a lot we can do …'

I was buggered if I knew what his problem was. But I could always get him set up on an IV-line to give me time to think and to reassure the others.

'Don't let him go, I'll try and find a vein and sedate him.'

Raoul tried to hold Gaston's hand still so I could inject him. Raoul was holding his arm so tight I thought I was ok and I wouldn't have to use a tourniquet. No such luck. Just as the needle of the catheter pierced his skin, Gaston had a sudden surge of energy and managed to rip everything out. Blood started to spurt. Here came the haematoma.

'Shit. Stop pissing around, Gaston! Calm down!'

'Jesus, Gaston, calm down,' added Raoul in his Savoyard accent.

Seeing as I was going to have to resort to strong-arm tactics, I took out my big sharp shiny scissors and cut through the sleeve. You can't beat the fold of the arm. The needle went straight into a big fat vein, as the blood flowing into the cannula demonstrated.

'Quick, a cap!'

Too late, I had blood all over my hands and I hadn't even put any gloves on. The syringe was almost ready.

'Hold on, guys, almost there!' I shouted.

The words had barely left my lips when Gaston started wriggling again. Raoul too: he got him in a headlock. But it was too late, he'd folded his arm. The cap had flown off with the catheter not far behind. Back to square one.

'That's enough, Gaston, just give it a rest, will you,' shouted Raoul.

'Get off me, you bastards. Help!' bellowed Gaston.

Alain said nothing. He had a crestfallen look about him.

I pitied Gaston. You could see the confusion, anxiety and terror in his face. What was going through his mind? He must have thought we were trying to torture him. I was racking my brain about what was wrong with him. This wasn't part of some kind of chronic hallucinatory psychosis, was it? Or maybe a tumour? After all, this wouldn't be the first time a tumour had shown up with the symptoms of hypoxia. Or why not a high-altitude cerebral oedema, the famous altitude sickness that makes people go mad? It is well known among Himalayan climbers and is often mentioned in the accounts by the great mountaineering pioneers.

There was the memorable case in South America, after I had just come down from Aconcagua in Argentina. My mate Nicolas and I had decided to make the ascent in under ten days. This was a stupid idea as all the texts you read on the subject, including the works to which I contribute, tell you to take your time when at altitude. Do as I say, not as I do …

It is all about respecting your ascent rate. Above 3,000 metres, the drop in air pressure is such that it takes the body time to organize itself and allow its various intracellular fluid compartments to readjust and produce more red blood cells. The body undergoes significant changes both physically and in terms of its metabolism. You just have to see the effects on a plastic bottle taken up to 5,000 metres, how much it expands and swells, to get an idea of what can happen to each and every one of the cells in our bodies.

We walked down from Aconcagua exhausted and naturally night had caught up with us. A multitude of dead-end paths taking us the wrong way meant we wasted a great deal of time. And two or three times we even wondered if we hadn't gone too low. The icy wind meant we didn't want to stop for any time at all, as we risked severe hypothermia. Our energy levels were well and truly exhausted and we were still at an altitude of 5,000 metres. Suddenly, as if by some kind of miracle, at two o'clock in the morning our minuscule tent appeared in the night. We had chosen it because it was so lightweight, with the idea of wandering all over Patagonia and Tierra del Fuego. It was microscopic, a kind of ambulatory sarcophagus. There was just enough room at the bottom for our feet and the front wasn't even high enough for us to crouch.

We were slumped in it like a couple of human wrecks. Neither of us had the wherewithal to boil any water. Our minds were already wandering halfway between nightmarish fantasies and a vague feeling of well earned serenity when, mixed in the noise of the wind, came the cries of an animal that had to be a Yeti ... Just as we had agreed by silent assent that it must have been a hallucination, the tent sank on top of us. Under the weight of a living mass.

'What's that?' screamed Nico.

'Hello.'

Silence.

It was a bloke. Probably one of the climbers we had seen arrive at base camp the day after our first acclimatization cycle at high camp.

He was jabbering away in what must have been German. We were wrapped up in our sleeping bags and it took us ten minutes of struggling to get out as the guy was slumped over our entrance. He was going to break everything.

He must have had a lot to tell us, given the amount of gibberish he was spouting. But he was in a pitiful state and we were freezing to death outside. Seeing as he had arrived out of nowhere and was in no fit state to go anywhere else, we would have to have him in with us. After a heroic effort, Nico and I managed to get him into our minuscule cabin. We squashed him in between the two of us so that he could make the most of the warmth from our sleeping bags. He still had his clothes and big boots on. For an instant, I thought we were finally going to be able to get some rest before first light. No such luck. Ten minutes later our lad started raving deliriously. We tried as best we could to reason with him but he was becoming violent and we didn't have any miracle pills to give him to reduce the oedema that was obviously squeezing his brain.

In the end he wriggled out of the tent and ran off into the night. Weary from our fight with the nutcase and because we were too knackered, we let him go. I spent the rest of the night regretting not stopping him and the guilt was still gnawing away at me the following morning. We weren't very proud of ourselves as we stuck our noses out of the tent. I saw Nico casting worried glances here and there, looking for a lifeless body.

It was only the following morning that we met our zombie again. It was he who came to find us, in the village where we had hired our mules. He was alive, and more incredible still was the fact that he recognized us. He thanked us and apologized for having disturbed us. I thought we had been pretty average on that count but he was convinced we had saved his life. We had a drink together. His name was Bergen and he had tried to get to his camp 2, above our camp. He too had been caught out in the maze of interlacing descent paths and, as he wasn't very well acclimatized at that stage, the night pretty much finished him off. He remembered fighting with us, then nothing, a complete blank. It was a miracle he managed to find his way, especially in the state he was in.

Gaston reminded me of the story. Cerebral oedema at this altitude? Unlikely. But what *did* he have?

Yet again I ended up going for the powerful option: Ketamine. I obviously like the drug. If I ever retrain I'm going to be a Ketamine drug rep! I knew very well that it was hardly recommended in these cases of psychosis but I didn't see how else we were going to deal with him, unless we just let him wreck everything in the helicopter. You don't stand a chance against a horse tranquilizer. Two minutes later, Gaston was rigid, completely disconnected from reality and his eyes staring as if he'd seen the devil himself. The tension eased off. Everyone could breath again, including Gaston. It was for the best. As the beast was now sleeping we tied him up in the stretcher. I quickly got a catheter into one of his veins to give him a bit of a sedative – midazolam – to prevent a bad trip when he woke up.

Alain relaxed, but what a palaver. His fifty-something client hadn't looked violent.

Raoul, who was watching Gaston, said to me, 'Look, Manu, your bloke's gone bright red.'

'No kidding, he's got enough layers on for a winter ascent, we could peel him like an onion.'

Something suddenly clicked in my mind. Bright red, no perspiration. I felt his forehead, his snout: he was burning up, you could almost fry an egg on him.

'I've got it. It's malignant hyperthermia! He must have a temperature of at least forty-one.'

The other two looked at me sceptically. Because I had used the word 'malignant' they were already thinking it was some kind of cancer. I was very pleased with myself and my diagnosis, and I was rushing around excitedly.

'We've got to cool him down. He's in a coma.'

So the three of us set about ripping his clothes off. With this kind of pathology, cooling him down as quickly as possible was the best treatment we could offer.

'Shame there isn't more snow, we could have shoved it under his arms and between his legs.'

The other two kept quiet and did as they were told. I decided to rehydrate him with some saline solution, otherwise he was going to shrivel up like a prune.

'We'll have to take him to intensive care. This kind of case will please Big Chief.' I couldn't stop myself from thinking out loud. Raoul and Alain gave me embarrassed looks.

'Well, it's true. He looked pretty depressed this morning, it gets him down when the beds are empty… Besides, it makes a change from hypothermia!'

I dithered about whether to get all the ironmongery out. I looked at Gaston: he was sedated, his blood pressure was good, if a little high. Thanks to the mask we'd put over his nose, his oxygen saturation was up to 95 per cent and we were at 2,000 metres. We were ready for a scoop and run. It was a three-minute flight to the hospital, where we could hand him over to Big Chief.

Big Chief wasn't there. The anaesthetist on call was Chaussée-aux-moines. He wasn't cut from the same mould as Big Chief. He was a nice guy, but whereas Big Chief was a bit too hands-on at times, Chaussée-aux-moines was quite the opposite. He got his nickname from his bald spot and was capable of anything, the very best work and the worst. We would get off lightly if he fancied working but that evening he had already slipped into his running shorts ready to go jogging. He really didn't want to have to get changed again.

I challenged him as I got out of the helicopter and as he was trying to make a quick getaway to his car to go running.

'It's back to work for you, granddad! I've brought you someone. A bit tricky, he can't be left on his own. You can kiss goodbye to your run this evening.'

He was trapped and had to wait for me to fill him in. We slid the rescue stretcher on to the hospital trolley while I told him about the patient.

'Better take his temperature. I'm sure he's suffering from malignant hyperthermia. He was completely delirious and he's burning up. Had to give him a shot of Ketamine. Had no choice. I'll pop by and see him this evening.'

We headed back to the DZ for another tidying up session. During the scrap, Gaston had managed to make a complete mess of my bag.

Alain came to see me as I was leaving at the end of the day. He looked a bit shaken up. The ice axe had left a gash on his forehead that needed stitches. I took him to get sewn up.

A&E looked like a battlefield after a battle. Nurses were running in all directions while the resuss room stank of puke and was being mopped down. Sandrine was white as a sheet. She never could stomach those kinds of smells and was spraying the room with lavender air-freshener. The atmosphere in the corridor confirmed that the late afternoon rush had been hard. As ever, they had nothing to do until four o'clock, when everyone arrived at once.

They had started off being brought an incontinent granny, referred by her GP and family, just before the weekend. What it really meant was that they wanted to get rid of her before going away for the weekend. On the doctor's letter, which was virtually illegible, there was no information about the treatment she was having or her medical history. We needed a bit of help as, obviously, no one from the family was with her and it was impossible to get hold of the GP as the surgery was closed for the holidays, '… for emergency cases dial 15', the French equivalent of 999.

Bruno, an intern, was battling with a decidedly sleazy-looking character who didn't smell too good either, the kind to have a beer in the morning, a Ricard at midday and an eau de cologne aperitif in the evening. I knew the guy, as he spent his time in A&E. There was always a scrap with him and it was draining work as he was phenomenally strong. He invariably ended up in the psychiatric hospital in La Roche-sur-Foron, having been given an injection in his arse. He would sober up the following morning when his mother, feeling guilty and for fear of what he might do, discharged him. I gave it a month before he would be up to his old tricks again.

A skinny woman was walking unsteadily down the corridor, leaning on her IV pole. Another one whose only means of expression was to pretend to commit suicide by taking ten Lexomils. These days, to be taken seriously, depressed people prefer to swallow sleeping pills. It lets them sleep for twenty-four hours and have a quick talk with a psychiatrist straight afterwards before having another crisis two weeks later.

All the mountain emergencies were piling into the waiting room: sprained ankles, sunburn, wasp stings. Wasps, they are a bit like the vipers: we get so many people coming in claiming to have known someone who died from a wasp sting. They make a beeline for A&E in a complete panic and there's nothing better for setting off an allergic reaction than stress!

The helicopter had brought in two lots of walkers covered in cuts, with their heads bashed up. There was also the unmistakable chest pain patient, requiring a coronary catheterization who was transferred to Annecy hospital, the departmental centre for interventional cardiology.

Room 2 was a mess and Chaussée-aux-moines had ended up intubating Gaston. It was a reflex action with these anaesthetists! Talking to patients wasn't their thing. A good dose of sedative and a tube for breathing and that was that.

I found a small spot where I could do Alain's two stitches myself. It was going to be much quicker that way. Alain was worried he had screwed up with his client and was uncomfortable. You often find this ambiguity among the guides towards their responsibilities. When it comes down to it, their job is very like our own. These days clients don't hesitate to complain when things don't go well. Much like the patient-doctor relationship, relations between clients and guides have soured over the past few years. As a guide and a doctor, I get the worst of both worlds, doubling my chances of ending up in court!

For guides, safety has become essential, sometimes at the expense of a spirit of adventure and discovery. My guide friends often come to me for information, wanting to know exactly what happened, from the medical point of view, in an accident. I feel like I'm an interface between the possible inquest the rescuer will be obliged to attend, and his or her possible responsibility. I try to stay neutral and that's not always easy, and is made all the more difficult by the affinity I feel towards the guides. I'm one of them, after all. I am also a great supporter of freedom of action in the savage arenas of the mountains. This is the difference between mountaineering and other sports. Yet I am also of the opinion that there must be limits. Clients are not objects, they must be treated with respect.

In the case of Gaston's accident, Alain was not at fault: malignant hyperthermia is rare and thus unforeseeable. Plus, Gaston was old enough to know that you take your jumper off when you are too hot.

What saddens me about this stupid world where there always has to be someone to blame, is that there will also always be someone who will say the guide screwed up and will find sufficiently convincing arguments to create suspicion.

Alain had a dressing on his head but it looked like this was the least of his worries. It was Gaston he was worried about. To set his mind at ease, I suggested we go and find out how he was getting on. But the spectacle of an intensive care unit is not designed to be reassuring.

'Don't worry, Alain, the tubes are just for show. He just needs a bit of rest. We have to help him for a few days.'

'Do you think he'll pull through without any after-effects?' he asked me timidly.

'Should do, yeah. His CK levels are through the roof, but that's normal, he must have lost a few muscle cells.'

'Ah, right ... What are the CK levels?'

'It's the level of enzymes in the muscle cells. They are released into the blood when cells break down for one reason or another ... Malignant hyperthermia for instance. The body's thermoregulation centre is in the brain and the situation got too much for it. The heat, excessive exercise, lack of training and dehydration meant he overheated. The body's thermostat started up its cooling processes, like sweating, to cool down.

But if you're wrapped up like an Eskimo you can't sweat normally and you start to burn up. In some people this manifests itself with heat stroke and most of the time this is fine, as they slow down what they are doing. But for some people it goes to their head and they don't know what they're doing any more. It makes them go mad and we have no idea why. Paradoxically, they overreact to it and become hyperactive ...'

'There's an alarm going off ...'

Indeed, the heart monitor alarm was going off. The duty nurse gently brushed past us to check it. I detected a glimmer of panic flash across Alain's face. Corinne replaced the pulse oxymeter that had slipped off Gaston's finger and the alarm stopped.

'Will his brain be ok?' asked Alain.

'Yes, problem is, it's the kidneys that suffer. When the cells break down they release myoglobin into the blood. That sometimes buggers them up and then you're on dialysis for the rest of your life.'

Alain had a long face. He didn't really like the kidney bit. He thanked me all the same before collecting Gaston's things and taking them to Lyon, where Gaston's wife was waiting for news.

A WALK IN THE PARK

• • • • • • • • •

At an altitude of 2,500 metres, a small flame was flickering. The candle was burning itself out. Not a breath of wind disturbed Stania's thoughts and daydreaming. She snuggled up to Marco, huddled in her down jacket with its patches. She found Mickey, his eyes gleaming in the candlelight, fascinating. He spoke in a whisper, telling them about his solitary travels.

Mickey had joined them late that evening. Marco vaguely recognized him but that was all. Mickey was famous for his solo adventures. He rarely climbed with other people. He wasn't emotionally disturbed or unsociable, he just liked the sense of freedom. He wasn't very physically impressive. He was considerably smaller than average with a slight stoop and long forearms that made him look a bit like a spider. He was a wiry little man from the mountains with big ears. That was no doubt how he came by the nickname 'Mickey'. He made a modest living working in a sports shop, which allowed him to organize his work around the weather forecast.

There were only three of them sleeping in the Fourche bivouac hut that night. The long routes in this part of the massif weren't very popular any more. Luckily, there was the Kuffner that still attracted a few mountaineers to the area. Stania had been expecting to see more people, especially with the great high-pressure weather system that was forecast for the week.

In the space of a few hours Stania had got some tall tales out of the introverted little man. He opened up a bit in the quiet and intimacy of the bivouac hut, responding to Marco's questioning and telling them about his terrifying solo climbs up icy gullies, each one more overhanging than the last. Listening to him, he must have almost died innumerable times and must have played all his jokers. Stania lapped it up.

Marco remained less convinced. He had agreed to let himself be dragged up the Brenva Spur, but it was to make her happy. Stania was Polish and since she was a little girl she had lived for the mountains. She was used to a precarious existence and had ended up finding sanctuary with Marco. They were perfectly matched; he earned a living as a designer with an unpretentious advertising agency and she made a bit of money working for various charities. The Brenva represented a serious undertaking for her. It is a long route, far from the standard beaten paths, following the southeast buttress of Mont Blanc and finishing up at the Col de la Brenva. You then have to follow the three Mont Blancs route back down to get to the Aiguille du Midi.

It was a leisurely saunter for Mickey. To listen to him, you'd have thought it was a walk in the park for him, training for some secret project.

They went to sleep under the hut's damp blankets.

Three in the morning. The snow crunched under their crampons as Stania led the way. Marco silently followed ten metres behind her, his eyes fixed on the pool of light from his head-torch catching the lines of sastrugi on the surface of the glacier. To reach the foot of the spur, you have to cross the start of the two branches of the Brenva glacier. This part of the route is not very dangerous and thoughts turn to other things, as it is the middle of the night. First digest your coffee then catch your breath.

Mickey had slipped out a good quarter of an hour before them. He had to be back in Chamonix that afternoon, he had promised his boss. Stania spotted the light from his little torch galloping off at least 300 metres in front of them.

Mickey had already settled into his brutish pace. He felt very light. Do it in record time, soaring over the Brenva, the power of his breathing, a sense of domination. The mountains were the only place he could express himself. Such a grand and awe-inspiring place, accessible to his slight frame. David and Goliath ran through his thoughts as he set off up the final bend leading to the bergschrund.

Then there was a sudden, ridiculous feeling of floating. A useless, impotent gesture, to try and grab hold of something in the emptiness. A flash, a violent pain in his ribs ... Then darkness.

Stania got up early the next morning. She felt a mixture of emptiness and anxiety. Marco was sound asleep. They had managed to catch the last lift down the afternoon before. They hadn't had any problems on the route, but it had been a bit long at the end. The climb back up the ridge to the cable car station was awful and it took every last ounce of energy they had left in them. Marco had cursed a bit before shutting up, suffering from the lack of oxygen.

The high-pressure weather system remained and the moon was still in its waxing phase. Ideal conditions to get back into the mountains and Stania was going through a hyperactive phase, ideas for routes flashing through her mind. Although still aching all over, she knew there were other projects just waiting to be done.

The hardest part would be convincing Marco. He liked exploring the mountains in a rather bucolic fashion. The effort he had made to accompany Stania was supposed to have earned him a well-earned truce.

Stania made the most of it that day by preparing her jams, as it was raspberry-picking time. Tomorrow she would go and buy a pair of proper crampons as hers were heavy and worn out. When you saw what was on the market these days – solid, lightweight crampons with quick-fit strap systems – it seemed silly not to have a pair!

I left the DZ early that evening. It was the end of the holidays and things were slowing down. The mechanic had decided to give Dragon a good clean and I made the most of the lull to slip back to Taconnaz: I had to practise the trumpet.

I only had two lines to learn but the problem was trying to find a quiet moment when I wouldn't burst everyone's eardrums.

Cécile and I had arrived at a compromise: I could play the trumpet to my heart's content while she played the hoover. But if the telephone went during this time, you couldn't be sure anyone would hear it.

'Manu … MANU! Telephone, it's the PGHM …'

She held out the receiver to me, impassive, while I carefully put my trumpet back in its case.

'Hello, Manu? It's J-B. Is this a bad time?'

'Yeah, I'm playing the trumpet …'

'Oh, right. Sorry. It's just that I wanted to let you know about tomorrow morning. We're looking for a guy who didn't come back from a route. It's a local bloke. Mickey, d'you know him?'

'Yeah, I see him at the climbing wall from time to time. He trains like a madman.'

'Well, he set off for the Brenva on his own. He was supposed to work yesterday afternoon and today. It was Salvetti, who owns the sport shop, who called to ask us to do a recce.'

'Now?'

'No, tomorrow at six. But we don't really know where he is. You can stay at home and we'll call you if we need you.'

'Ok. Let's do that.'

There was no way I was going to get my trumpet practice done. I'd already missed my lesson the week before. I had to practise a little bit for the following day, else my teacher, Alex who was a good head taller than me, was going to give me a right earful.

I got the instrument out again, thinking about what would happen next. It was always the same in this kind of situation: either the chopper would come back empty-handed as the guy we were looking for had managed to get down under his own steam without telling anyone, or we would pick up a frozen body a few weeks, months or even years later.

That evening, after having read a few pages of my thriller, I had difficulty nodding off as I thought about the little guy full of energy who was wandering around goodness knows where in the mountains. I had few illusions as to his fate. I was worried we would find him stiff as a board at the bottom of the spur.

It was as if someone had bored an ice pick into his back. An electric shock shook him from head to toe, his whole body contorted in pain.

Mickey emerged from his nightmare. He felt the blade of a windscreen scraper along the length of his spine. The guy doing it was taking perverse pleasure in pushing the edge of it into him to make it even more painful.

He was lying in darkness between two blocks of ice. When he tried to roll over to get away from the windscreen scraper, he felt a stabbing pain in his chest. He was winded and let out a silent cry that was no comfort at all. Little by little the desperate reality of the situation came to him. He opened his left eye, the other remained glued shut. Two walls rose up around him like icy vaulting. He was lying on his back. His torn pack was wrapped around his head. Perhaps it had cushioned his fall. He was in tremendous pain around his pelvis. How long had he been there?

It came back to him. He remembered the night in the hut with Marco and Stania and the crunch of the glacier beneath the moon. Then there was the crevasse that he only saw at the last moment, his desperate attempt to place his ice axe, followed by the interminable fall. Everything was going so well, what an idiot. He was alone in a crevasse in a part of the massif where nobody went. Why hadn't the other two, behind him, seen what had happened? He imagined the couple roped together, carefully avoiding the crevasse, just like you're told to in all the good mountaineering books.

Daylight feebly shone through the ceiling of snow above. It must have been late in the day but he had no notion of time. He was suddenly overcome by an urgent need to pee. At least that seemed to be working ok. Mickey realized quite how bad he was as he tried to relieve himself. Undoing his fly demanded a fiendish amount of energy and an acceptance of more pain than he thought was actually possible. These trousers weren't built for poor blokes like him, who were in the middle of snuffing it!

He had to take stock of the situation, get out of his uncomfortable position and think. And, looking on the bright side of things, he had all the time in the world for that. Danger in the mountains is more often than not characterized by stressful situations requiring quick reactions and, if possible, the right decision. Everything happens in a few fractions of a second, a hand hold breaks, the rope snaps, an avalanche is triggered … It is all a question of fate and of primary reflexes. It was different for him, at the bottom of the crevasse. This was the other side of danger, its cold and unshakable opposite. The harm had been done, it was irreversible. The sentence had been delivered, and Mickey with it, into the jaws of the crevasse.

The gloomy walls of ice were insensible to his tears, to his cries for help, insensible to his suffering and reflected back to him nothing more than his already forgotten image.

Mickey felt sick as he considered the slow agony awaiting him. No, it wasn't over. He had to try something. He cried out in pain as he sat up. His pelvis was torture and his leg wasn't responding any more. Oh my God, he thought, I'm paralysed on one side.

He sat there crying for a few minutes. Then he felt pins and needles crawling up his thigh. He tried to move it. It works! He could move his thigh. He wasn't paralysed after all. At last, some good news, a glimmer of hope.

Mickey managed to prop up his back a bit better and drew up an inventory of the damage: a cut on his head that had stuck his hat to his hair, a few possible broken ribs, definitely a fractured pelvis and multiple bruises that he preferred not to think about.

Miraculously, he had held on to his gloves and his arms seemed to be working. Pushing himself along on his hands like some kind of legless cripple, he managed to extricate himself from the icy cubby-hole in which he was embedded. It was time to make a clearer evaluation of the situation. It reminded him of another story. Although he was hardly a fan of Herzog-style mountain dramas, he had let himself be dragged by a friend to see *Touching The Void* some time before. Lucky guy, Joe Simpson, it wasn't often there was a way out at the bottom of a crevasse. In any case, it wasn't looking good for him. He had a good look at the ground beneath him and it looked more like a mousetrap than an escape route to freedom. On the other hand, the crevasse, into which he had had the bright idea to fall, was not all that deep. The problem was the walls were overhanging.

Mickey needed a few hours to rest and prepare. He then set off up the ice, determined to squeeze out of his tomb. He had managed to salvage three ice screws but his ice axe was still in the lip of the crevasse, ten metres higher up. That would teach him to never use the leashes.

He had a searing pain in his ribs. At the slightest turn of his upper body, he felt a crushing pain all over his chest, which stopped him breathing. He had been given a foretaste of what to expect when, in a flash of lucidity, he had pounced on his backpack to get his mobile. It was still in one piece and charged but he had no bars. At the bottom of a crevasse the other side of Mont Blanc, it would have been too good to be true! His broken ribs instantly manifested themselves. He let out a great cry and then waited five minutes to get his breath back.

He made a kind of étrier with two slings to move up from one ice screw to another. He had worked out a very simple technique: place an ice screw as high as possible, clip himself to it with a sling, place another screw just below it to attach his etrier. He pulled himself up on to this one using the less painful of his legs, stood up and placed his third ice screw higher up. He then had to hang from the highest one to undo the lowest of the screws before starting the process over again. It was child's play, as long as you had good ice and your pelvis was in good nick. Mickey got started. His watch said three in the afternoon. How could he have been unconscious for so long? No doubt it was what the docs called a coma.

He had to get out before nightfall. It seemed doable. Once he was out, he'd go and shelter in the Fourche hut, dragging himself along. There was a chance he'd pull through.

Placing the first ice screw quickly brought him to his senses. The ice was blue and glassy and as hard as steel. Simply pushing on the ice screw as he tried to turn it was excruciating. Two hours later he still hadn't even managed to clip himself to the second screw. He was covered in sweat, as the work required a superhuman effort from him. Night was falling and Mickey hadn't even climbed three metres. It was torture hanging in the harness. It was almost unbearable.

Nevertheless, after several hours of toil, Mickey had reached the upper part of the wall. The glassy grey appearance of the ice left him in no doubt as to its mediocre quality. And the overhang was getting steeper. All of a sudden, as he placed the next screw, pushing even harder with his wrist, the whole plate of ice cracked with a dull noise. Mickey carried on turning the screw in the hope that it would bite underneath, but the ice came away and took out the screw attached to his foot loop. Mickey fell backwards into space, head first. He heard the bones in his pelvis creak at the same time as he nearly passed out with pain. Fuck, that's it, I'm going to die, he thought, resigned to his fate. He waited for the final screw to pull out. The fucker's holding! What's going on? The one that was supposed to hold ripped, and the one that wasn't supposed to hold stayed in!

The bit of rope he had tied to the back of his harness to attach his bag was dangling in front of his eyes. In a final desperate effort, he made a loop and clipped it to the last ice screw, which was holding everything. He made an Italian hitch on the karabiner on his harness and hurriedly set about lowering himself down before the whole thing ripped and he crashed to the ground, four metres below. The hardest part was unclipping the sling he was attached to from the ice screw. The pain was so great that, if he had had a knife in his hand, he wouldn't have thought twice about cutting the lot. In the meantime, to give himself some slack, he had no other choice but to grab one of the ice screws that was dangling below and screw it back in. He could then put his weight back on this one, unclip himself from the top ice screw and lower himself down to the ground.

He collapsed to the ground like a dead weight. He wanted to be sick but there was nothing left in his stomach. A wave of cold sweat ran down his face. He saw the crevasse spinning around his head in the half-light. An icy shudder ran down his body and he lapsed once more into unconsciousness.

Stania tripped on the carpet and almost squashed a Japanese man who was trying to leave. She apologized, a bit embarrassed. The Japanese man replied with a respectful bow.

The footwear and crampon department was in the basement. She knew exactly what she wanted: Grivels with quick-fit straps. That's what Mickey had recommended. Plus they were in the sale and it was the time to make the most of the end of the season.

Apparently Mickey wasn't there. She would have liked to have heard how the route had gone two days before.

Bruno came up to her. He normally worked on the floor above.

'Hi, Stania. How's it going?' he asked a little distractedly.

'Hi, Bruno.'

'You looking for something?'

'Yeah, some crampons, the Grivel ones. Mickey told me they were in the sale.'

'Oh yeah, we should have a few pairs left.'

'Mickey's not here, is he?' she ventured.

'Don't you know?'

'Know what?'

'No one knows where he is. He didn't come back from his climb the day before yesterday. He didn't come to work yesterday and he still hasn't been in this morning. Salvetti called the PGHM. They looked all over for him this morning but no one knows where he's got to.'

'Mickey? But I was with him the day before yesterday. He was going to do the Brenva. I was climbing with Marco.'

Twenty minutes later Stania turned up at the PGHM. A woman was coming out, her face drawn and her eyes red.

When Stania told the gendarme what she knew, he rushed over to catch the girl leaving. She was Mickey's girlfriend. Stania had never met her before. She had an unassuming and shy look about her. There was a glimmer of hope in her eyes as she looked at Stania. Mickey hadn't even told her where he was going.

Now they had to work out where he might have vanished.

Thinking back, Stania had been a little concerned not to see Mickey above them once dawn had come. The long snow and ice ridge leading to the Col de la Brenva was visible from the glacier. Even as they started up the bottom section of the ridge they should have been able to see him on the crest. You can normally see people climbing the Brenva for the length of the route, up to the séracs at the top. In the end, Stania had told herself that Mickey was really going well and was already at the top.

Stania tried to recall the possible traps he might have encountered. On the walk in, there was only a single crevasse blocking the route before the first little col. She and Marco had carefully gone round underneath it. She didn't remember seeing any tracks that finished abruptly in the middle of it. It hadn't snowed for ten days and the glacier was dry. Mickey could have slipped at the top, where the ridge was most icy. But there were so many other places, on the descent, where he could have been swallowed up in a hole.

'Come in, Dragon, this is Cordial.'

'Yes, Cordial, we're listening,' replied Jean, the mechanic.

'Don't put the chopper away yet, you've got another recce to do.'

'Don't worry if it's for the guy who works at Salvetti's, we've already spent ages looking. Unless you've got some more info, we can't do very much. We can't trawl through the whole Mont Blanc Massif.'

'Yep, we've got some new info. There's someone who saw him setting off for the Brenva. I'll call you on the TPH.'

TPH stands for telephone. When it comes to giving detailed information, we try to avoid using the emergency channel as a number of people in Chamonix are permanently tuned in to it. There are all sorts: those passionate about rescues, those nostalgic for the old days, voyeurs, and prats who will go round spreading any kind of gossip. There are even some who find it entertaining to set off a false alarm. I remember one guy who managed to mobilize around ten or so rescuers and cause two days of searching with the helicopter at over 4,000 metres by falsely claiming to be in trouble somewhere near the Montagne de la Côte, below the summit of Mont Blanc. By the time we had managed to bring in the specialist equipment from Lyon to locate the crafty little sod, the calls had stopped.

Hence it is customary only to give out the bare minimum of information over the airwaves and certainly not to mention any names.

The rescue gendarme on duty, Benoît 'Ben' Debraise, took the matter in hand. He had curly hair and big honest blue eyes. As soon as a delicate situation comes up, his pugnacious spirit is awakened and he is ready to move mountains to save widows and orphans. Besides, he has a soft spot for pretty girls. It was he who collected Stania and took her to the DZ.

At eight in the evening as the sky was darkening and the massif turned red, Dragon took off to fly over the Brenva

Spur. Yvon, the pilot, didn't hold out much hope but he had eaten a good sandwich, there was a beautiful sunset and he had nothing against staying a bit later. Yvon had never been a high-level mountaineer. Half of him felt a sense of admiration while the other half was dismayed when he watched the foolish kids setting off all around him for hard routes on their own. He was a father himself. The mere thought of freezing his arse off during the annual survival courses he had to do was enough to leave him with absolutely no desire to wander around the mountains in any way other than at the controls of his helicopter.

Stania was excited. She had an ambiguous feeling, she was torn between the fun of flying over the massif at sunset and anxious that they would find Mickey lifeless at the bottom of the ridge. She couldn't believe it. For the first time in her life she was getting into a helicopter yet it might also be the first time she would come face to face with death.

The four occupants of the Alouette scrutinized every detail of the spur. Yvon flew low over the foot of the other side of the east buttress. He even swung past the start of the Voie Major, in case Mickey had changed route at the last minute.

The night was beginning to cast its shadows over the whole area. At Stania's request, Yvon hovered one last time over the small crevasse before the start of the route. As they studied the gaping wound in the ice, they all had the same thought and it was Ben who spoke first.

'We better have a look in the hole tomorrow morning. It's in the middle of the track. What do you think, Stania?'

'I agree. In the dark the other morning we could have easily fallen into it,' she replied with her faint East European accent.

'Right, let's go home. In any case, I can't see a thing and I'm out of fuel. Take off at 6 a.m. tomorrow with all the gear,' declared Yvon.

I was watching cartoons with the kids … I hadn't got much done that day. It was the kind of day where you either get everything done or nothing goes right. Millions of things to do, thousands of promises to keep, but it was impossible to know where to start. I had wandered between the hospital, the DZ and the house, trying to sort out work for the next month and reply to the fifty-three emails that had been sitting in my inbox for the past three days. There were a lot of requests for courses with helicopters, questions about acute mountain sickness from those leaving on expedition, articles to correct and dozens of those bloody adverts that I never seem to be able to get rid of.

Dragon had flown around in the mountains looking for the famous Mickey. But there was no news. No kidding! They were hoping to find the man in a five-kilometre wide chain of mountains stuffed full of pitfalls. They may as well have been looking for a bacterium in a block of ice.

Ben called me at eight at night to let me know they had some information on Mickey. A Polish woman had met him at the Fourche hut. He was going to do the Brenva Spur before going down to work that afternoon. Dragon had done another reconnaissance flight that evening without success. The rescuers were going to be dropped off the following morning to look in the crevasse at the start of the climb, in the middle of the approach route. I would be ready but I didn't see what I was going to be able to do for someone who had spent the last three days in a crevasse.

In these cases, if we can't save lives, we recover the bodies. We sometimes end up in impossible situations. Some families are prepared to spend a fortune to bring back the body of a dead loved one. I witnessed this kind of determination when a boy I knew was swallowed up by a crevasse in Bolivia. More than fifty Andean villagers were drafted in to climb a mountain of over 5,000 metres to extract his body trapped seventeen metres below the surface of the glacier. The family was very persuasive but it had endangered the lives of the poor villagers for a pittance.

ALIVE

· · · · · · · · ·

In the crevasse, Mickey was shaking uncontrollably. He was struggling with the guy who wouldn't stop pestering him. 'Up you get, Mickey, you're bloody useless. It's not the gear's fault, it's your fault … No, it's all right. I'm kidding. Ooh, listen, can you hear that buzzing? I know that noise …' He flitted around between the sky and the ground, and the ice and snow.

The buzzing woke him up. He knew that noise. He had to hold on. It would be easy just to fall asleep and surrender himself to the great white hand clasping him. It would be so relaxing not to be in pain, not to be moving any more. You can't give up. He knew that. He had read it in all the mountain books he had devoured: if you fall asleep the white devil will take you away for eternity. Hallucinations hammered away at his mind. He saw himself in the hands of faceless scientists, his body frozen in a lump of ice and donated to science. They tried defrosting him. He saw himself covered in hair with the features of an orang-utan. The slightest movement of his pelvis, the smallest touch of his fingers set off great spasms of pain.

The noise of the rotor blades drifted away. It was much easier just to fall back into a torpor.

Damn that bloody ringing. Six-thirty. Cécile reached the phone first. It was her bright idea to keep it on her side of the bed.

'Yeah, hello?... Yep, I'll hand you over.'

She handed the thing to me and went back to sleep.

'Yeah?' I grumbled.

'Up you get, Manu! They found Mickey this morning. He's at the bottom of a slot. You've got to come to the DZ, they're waiting for you to go up again.'

'Is he alive?'

'I've no idea.'

I jumped into my trousers and flew down the stairs, trying not to miss the last steps. I hate being rushed early in the morning. Luckily I had had the good sense to prepare my stuff the night before. There wasn't a breath of wind and it was absolutely calm outside. The freshness of the morning stung my nostrils. The car juddered and spluttered before starting.

'Get a move on, Manu. They're waiting for you.'

Jean, the mechanic, was raring to go. Just like his chopper, he was clean and immaculately turned out. The helicopter was already warm and ready to climb up into the icy heights.

I couldn't help marvelling at the beauty of the landscape. It never fails to be spectacular. The Grandes Jorasses were silhouetted in the background, their needles of rock bristling towards the spreading dawn. The light of the new day was blending into the red glow over the Envers du Mont Blanc. Its slopes wearily warmed themselves in the first rays of sun, while the great red insect buzzed the procession of crevasses lined up and facing the same way. Forbes bands cut across the ribbon of the Mer de Glace as it fled downwards, disappearing into the darkness of the silent valley below. The glacier in the

Combe Maudite awaited us and the engine slowed down. We made a few turns, brushing past the Grand Capucin and the buttresses of the Tour Ronde, gaining enough height to finally cross the Col de la Fourche.

The ants were there, red and blue against the snow, bustling around the tiny open wound in the snow. I got out.

'More … More … Stop,' I said.

'Ok, I've got you,' replied Jack in the walkie-talkie.

'Look out. Got to get the static line out of the way. It's caught in the lip.'

'What?'

'Flip up the static line. It's going to bring the cornice down. Give it some slack and flip it out of the way.'

'Got it. Ok,' crackled the walkie-talkie.

The white rope went slack and was jerked.

I let myself be lowered down into the slot, suspended from a cable a few millimetres thick and clutching the stretcher. I was already cut off from the surface and plunged on into another world, the great icy blue.

I found Ben at the bottom of the chasm, looking up at me. He had placed a couple of ice screws in the wall, to which he had clipped himself. A body lay at his feet, not moving …

'He's cold. I'd even say he was frozen. What do you think, Ben?'

Ben stared at me intently, as if his own fate depended on it.

'So you don't think he's dead then? I was right to get you to come?' he said excitedly.

'Yes, well done. There isn't much we can do for him but it wouldn't take much to finish him off either.'

Even as I spoke, I wondered how I could have trotted out such nonsense. Then again, there was some sense in what I was saying. Mickey was rigid, his arms and legs stiff and motionless. He wasn't talking any more and appeared to have stopped breathing. I put two fingers under his nose and I thought I could sense his furtive breathing. This was a simple yet effective technique that I had put to the test over the years. The skin on the back of your fingers is equipped with numerous heat-sensitive receptors. I have yet to find a better way of telling if someone is breathing or not. In hypothermia cases, the body slows down, the pulse rate, respiratory rate and volume decrease. When the body's temperature drops to 25 degrees, the oxygen consumption in cells is half the normal level. The cardio-pulmonary system, which provides the energy vital for the body's organs, reduces its work rate thanks to the intervention of an ingenious system of control.

Mickey was breathing of his own accord, he was alive, a little smashed up, but alive.

I grabbed the mini heart monitor and pulse oxymeter to confirm what I hoped was true.

'Here, Ben, put that on the end of his finger.'

For my part, I tried to open the top of Mickey's jacket to slide in the electrodes for the heart monitor. It's an ingenious little device that is designed for these kinds of situations. Metal patches placed on the right parts on the chest plot the heart's electrical activity on a screen. The image is not particularly high quality but it is good enough. Spikes showed a regular ventricular contraction of thirty beats per minute.

'It's not working, Manu, it just keeps flashing,' said Ben, trying to get the blood-oxygen saturation of Mickey's blood with the device on the end of his finger.

'Leave it, Ben. His hands are too cold for it to work. Get out the tympanic thermometer.'

The infrared digital pulse oxymeter indicates the oxygenation levels in the blood but if, for one reason or another, the blood flow has slowed it can be difficult to read.

I continued my auscultation of Mickey, trying to assess the extent of the damage. He couldn't have fallen that far without breaking something. Mickey wasn't even wearing a helmet. He was obviously one of those unorthodox climbers who preferred placing his life in the hands of fate, the kind of people who think a helmet is an unnecessary weight offering poor protection against the forces of evil! We later found Mickey's helmet in the bottom of his pack ...

Broken ribs, that was for sure. Crevasse accidents always cause broken ribs. It remained to be seen if they had pierced his lungs. In that case, warming him up could be a complex procedure. In my mind, I drew up a list of Mickey's possible injuries upon which his fate would hang. I normally start from the head and work my way down. This means I don't have to think too hard when I'm in an environment that doesn't lend itself to great intellectual deliberation. Skull, lungs, intra-abdominal haemorrhaging with the classic ruptured spleen, pelvis, and femurs ... I always finish up by checking the cervical-spine alignment and test the motor functions and sensitivity of the legs to make sure there are no major spinal injuries. Obviously, Mickey couldn't be asked.

I helped Ben place the thermometer in Mickey's ear. The thermometer was the work of a Swiss engineer from the canton of Vaud. All specialists know that a person's core temperature can be taken in different ways and that the most reliable readings are those taken nearest the heart. This is entirely based on empirical evidence and is a source of much discussion in the scientific community. Some think that it is the cerebral temperature that determines the main variations in the adaptation mechanisms and not that of the heart. Currently, it is readings obtained by intracardiac catheterization that are considered the standard reference values. It goes without saying, that it is impossible to take these kinds of readings in an emergency situation. Similar readings, obtained using rectal and oesophagus thermometers, are used to aid an initial diagnosis in hospitals. But it is hard to see yourself stripping patients in the snow to shove a tube up their backsides. Equally, passing the same kind of probe into the stomach, via the nose or clamped mouth, of a hypothermia victim would be as great a challenge. Although the results are less precise, Monsieur Métraux's tympanic thermometer remains our only option.

I peered at the digital reading on the small liquid crystal screen as it slowly rose. It settled at 23.4 degrees.

'Twenty-three degrees! Is that possible?' asked Ben.

'Yep, it's possible. That tallies with his clinical state.'

'Is that serious? What happens next?'

'We don't get worked up and try not to screw up. We've got to sort ourselves calmly. I need the stretcher and the KED and a chopper on stand-by for Geneva.'

'Ok. I'll call them.'

I looked at Mickey, I was amazed how tough he was: three nights in a crevasse after the fall he had taken! In a way, this proved he wasn't suffering from any 'major injuries liable to compromise the overall prognosis', as emergency doctors would have it. His main problem was hypothermia. We were going to have to get him out of there as gently as possible, to make sure his heart didn't stop. At this stage of hypothermia, the slightest stimulation could have brought on heart failure. By a simple mistake while handling him …

Beyond that of Christ, literature is full of miraculous resurrections that defy explanation. There was one recently that was the subject of a very serious paper, which challenged us all. While crossing a valley on a ski trip, a young Scandinavian woman was caught unawares and fell into a crevasse. By sheer luck and thanks to the shape of the hole beneath her, in which there was a fast-flowing glacial torrent, she found herself wedged, with her head in the air and her body submerged. She still had her skis on and they were caught under her, which made getting her out difficult. It took her friends more than ninety minutes to free her. Her heart had stopped beating. Her friends had good first-aid skills and gave her heart massage until she was taken to the A&E department of a teaching hospital. When she was taken into the resuss room her core temperature was 13.7 degrees, and her heart was already in cardiac arrest. One hundred and sixty minutes had already gone by.

The young woman was taken to a heart surgery unit and was warmed up on a machine providing extracorporeal circulation.

At this time, the ECC is the best means of quickly warming hypothermia victims. We can gain five degrees every hour. To the amazement of everyone concerned, the Norwegian woman's heart was restarted with a defibrillator once her temperature reached 30°C.

Listening to Gordon, one of the most eminent Canadian specialists in the field, tell the story in a lecture and while watching the video of the young woman in question talking candidly about the accident and admitting she must have used quite a few of her nine lives that day, I wondered grimly how many victims we had buried alive …

Mickey's arms were rigid and I couldn't see any obvious veins. I preferred not to try and get an IV-line going. In any case, at that moment in time what good would it have done? I'd have been hard pressed to do anything much as I was suspended over nothing while we were bringing him back up to the surface.

I chose to be winched up with Mickey to protect him from being knocked around. We carefully wrapped him up in the KED with a cervical collar and the mini heart monitor whose electrodes I had already attached to his chest. I had my eyes glued to the cable in front of me, and was surprised to find myself praying as we were silently lifted up towards the heavens.

As ever, the trickiest moment was getting over the lip of the crevasse but Mickey was holding on.

'Manu, Dragon went off for a femur while you were in the hole. I've scrambled Fox for Geneva. Is that still OK with you?' asked Jack as I took off my crampons.

'Shit, that's not good. I really needed Dragon.'

'Yes, but they're likely to need you for the femur. What are we doing with Mickey?'

'Hang on, give him some oxygen. While you do that, I'll call Arnold. He should have his gear with him. He can go to Geneva. Shit, no network … Bollocks.'

'Use Cordial to call him,' suggested Jack.

'I've got no choice. I hate it when it's complicated, half the info gets lost on the way.'

I contacted Cordial by radio to pass on a short but comprehensive report to Arnold.

The trickiest bit would be contacting 15 to explain we wanted a bed in Geneva. We had spent a great deal of energy, a while before, establishing a protocol for transferring our hypothermia cases to the cantonal hospital in Geneva. It is the only unit within an hour of Chamonix with an ECC machine. To have a chance of saving our patients, we had to make a request direct to the heart surgery department, which had assured us of its support. Arnold had put a great deal of effort into the system. I knew he would ensure the transfer went smoothly.

In the meantime, I was stuck there. Since I had to wait, I may as well do something. Seeing as we were no longer in the bottom of a crevasse, I set about getting an IV-line going. I injected Mickey with 250 millilitres of saline solution that was still warm from having been in the bottom of my pack. I couldn't have given him fluids that risked cooling him down even more! Plus, it's useful to know that a few pieces of Cordura stitched together will maintain a bit of heat. I thanked the heavens I had brought my gear into the house the night before.

IN DOCTORS' HANDS

• • • • • • • • •

Arnold was getting annoyed.

'You've got two choices: either you do as I tell you or you leave, but don't come crying to us when you get carted off tonight because you're paralysed down one side.'

'Piss off! I'm free to go home. I'm not a kid any more,' replied the tanned man in his sixties.

Victor Bardeluc, the former marketing manager for the Bluesky laboratories, was on holiday in his chalet in Les Praz and wasn't used to being given orders.

Arnold came back with, 'Exactly, you're not a kid any more, so be reasonable!'

Arnold was at the top of his game that day. He had arrived in a rush that morning, already on the go. It was his third day on duty and the night had been hard. He had been disturbed by injured alcoholics throughout the night and hadn't been able to get any rest.

By nine in the morning, after having drunk two strong coffees, he had thrown A&E into chaos. Nurses were running right, left and centre trying to sort out the directions for treatment he had already changed at least twice. Five people were back in the waiting room for dressings and sprained ankles from the day before. Two people were making a nuisance of themselves, having a go at the secretary, trying to get their documents and asking for certificates. The telephone was ringing off the hook and the whole team was ready to snap.

Fortunately, Simon, the second duty A&E doctor was a calm sort of chap, very calm in fact. He coolly started his rounds, completely indifferent to the mayhem around him. He patiently listened to the ravings of the female patient in cubicle 2, who had been brought in that night. He might have drifted off if Martine hadn't shaken him awake. Yet the advantage of his imperturbability was that it offset Arnold's rising blood pressure, as he had decided not to let his patient go.

The discussion had started with strong words. Victor Bardeluc had been brought in by his wife and daughter who had found him haggard and drawn at the foot of the bed. He looked at them, lost, unable to remember what he had done for the previous three days. His face was lopsided and the corner of his mouth was turned down. It gave him a world-weary look his wife hadn't seen before.

In Arnold's case, it was his glasses that were crooked. The more agitated he got, the more lopsided they became. Add to that his shaggy hair and you've got the perfect look for getting your patient on your side.

Nadia would have liked to have interrupted him for thirty seconds to ask which blood tests needed to be done on the patient in the cubicle next door, given that Arnold hadn't input anything into the computer. But she couldn't get a word in edgeways. The young Pole was just passing through and came in with a raging sore throat and Arnold suspected he was carrying avian flu. Arnold had recently got back from Thailand and suspected everyone of having it.

Bardeluc had stood up to get dressed. He had decided to leave the hospital.

'Listen to me! Lie down and listen to me,' Arnold insisted.

No reaction.

'Will you listen to me, Monsieur Bardeluc!' he said again, getting irritated.

'Listen to him, dear,' chimed in Madame Bardeluc.

'Listen to the doctor. They need to do some ad-dition-al tests,' she said slowly, sighing.

Victor Bardeluc lay back down, grumbling.

'Arnold, the patient next door has got a temperature of 40.3 degrees. What should I do?' Nadia finally managed to ask.

'Ah, yes, he is hot!' said Arnold delightedly in a professorial tone.

'Arnold, the PGHM are coming to pick you up. You've got to get ready to take a hypothermia case to Geneva.'

'Balls! I've got my hands full here!'

Nadia looked at him powerlessly.

'It's Manu who got them to call you. They've got two rescues at once.'

'So how's Manu's hypothermia victim?'

'I don't know. It was the PGHM that told me.'

'What's his temperature? Is he injured?'

'I told you I don't know. Call them back!'

'Right, Simon will have to take over here. I've just convinced Bardeluc to stay to have his scan. I won't be happy if he does a runner. He doesn't look like a patient man!'

'You can talk!'

Arnold was already thinking about the rescue operation and, letting the remark go, dropped what he was doing and rushed off to the phone.

'Hello? Yeah, what's the story? ... It's Arnold!'

The gendarme at the other end of the line must have asked who the man barking down the phone at him was.

'Where? At the bottom of the Brenva ... How much? Twenty-three degrees ... Is he in cardiac arrest?... You have no idea ... What? Chopper, in five minutes. Right, ok.'

Arnold hung up and looked distractedly at Nadia.

'Shit! I forgot to ask if the CODIS had been alerted. Well, they must have. The other helicopter was scrambled ...'

The CODIS was the departmental operation centre for fires and rescues, which had to be alerted when transport was being arranged from one sector to another, in this case from Chamonix to Geneva.

Nadia tried to follow, by a process of deduction, Arnold's thought processes. She didn't understand everything but as he was asking the questions and giving the answers ...

'Right. I'll call Geneva myself,' he decided all of a sudden.

When it comes to persuading people to do things, Arnold is a master, and he could sell ice creams on an iceberg. In five minutes it was in the bag.

'They'll take him!' he cried victoriously.

But as he was running to the office he suddenly stopped and turned to Nadia with a look of panic on his face.

'Shit! I haven't got my gear ...'

Arnold had found a helmet: it was one of Big Chief's. As were the glasses he had crookedly plonked on top of his head. He had dug out an old harness and Gore-Tex jacket that were hanging round the office. It would be fine, he probably wouldn't even have to get out of the chopper. He had knicked a pack of medical gear from the paramedics.

The chopper had just picked him up and he tried to control his excitement by watching the vertiginous ridges of the pillars on the east face of the Tacul as they raced past him. It was impressive how fast the EC 145 gained height. A far cry from the Alouette. They could already see the north face of the Tour Ronde appearing in the left-hand corner.

'Come in, doc, Fox calling.'

'Yep, I can hear you.'

I heard the drone of the big bumble-bee coming up towards us. It must have been the mechanic calling me.

'Arnold would like some more info about your patient.'

'Right. Hypothermia, his temperature's 23 degrees, his heart's beating. Associated injuries to chest and perhaps pelvis. In a crevasse for two days. He's got a GCS of five, I haven't intubated him.'

GCS was a coma scale, starting at 3 for brain dead and going up to 15, normal.

'Right, we'll take him as he is and head for Geneva straight away.'

'Ok, fine, we're ready.'

Two minutes later the great bumble-bee was right above our heads. A tornado of white froze us where we stood. Mickey was shoved inside like a pizza in an oven, quicker than we could even get the words out. The white tornado disappeared as quickly as it had appeared. The din died down and we were alone again. They'd stolen our patient!

Half an hour later, Fox touched down on the roof of the Geneva cantonal hospital. A Swiss doctor had joined the hospital porters to meet the patient. Arnold leapt out. Mickey had held on during the flight but he had hardly warmed up at all. So as not to risk an after drop, they were mindful not to put the heating on in the chopper. It was still a miracle Mickey had not gone into cardiac arrest.

The gigantic Swiss hospital looked every bit the part and was obviously well funded. Mickey was slid on to a well oiled hospital trolley and gently wheeled to the resuss room where a team of switched on emergency medicine technicians was waiting for him. There was a coordinating doctor, two anaesthetists, three nurses, a radiologist, an intern and two porters. When comparing our establishment in Chamonix with its Swiss counterpart, we jokingly remark that there are ten of them for one patient, and in Chamonix there is one of us for ten patients. That's where the famous couplet 'all for one and one for all' comes from! In the Geneva cantonal hospital, everyone has a job: there's the IV person, one for the ultrasound, a person for the intubation, someone to put a drain in, the person who does the urinary catheterization, the person who does the x-rays, and someone to write everything down and sort out the admission. It's much easier if there are ten of you. Unfortunately, it doesn't mean they're infallible ...

Arnold walked into the room with one of the rescuers. The contrast between the two was striking: his helmet was still sitting lopsidedly on his head, the just-out-of-the-mountains look. Thankfully, he had remembered to take his crampons off.

There was an air of Swiss calm in the room and Arnold introduced his patient.

'... Young mountaineer found in a crevasse after two days of looking, hypothermia, temperature of 23 degrees, but heart rate of 35 ...'

While he was speaking the team got into place to lift the patient off the trolley. Arnold continued, 'He's probably got some fractured ribs and we think the pelvis is broken too.'

They cut the clothes off Mickey.

'... Head wound but no means of doing a neurological exam ...'

They hooked him up to all the various machines: ECG, oxygen saturation levels, heart monitor, rectal thermometer ...

Arnold had to stop what he was saying as he was in the way. He left the resuss room with the rescuer to gather their equipment and oxygen bottle. But when he went back in he looked on in amazement. They had started cardiac massage.

'What are you doing?' exclaimed Arnold, astounded.

'Major bradycardia, no pulse, blood pressure in his boots,' replied the young anaesthetist, his eyes glued to the heart monitor.

Arnold was speechless.

'No choice,' added the Swiss doctor.

Arnold felt the blood throbbing in his ears. He was seeing red.

'But that's normal, he's got a temperature of 23 degrees! Blood pressure is always really low at that temperature. The one thing you don't do is give him cardiac massage, you're going to kill him!' he shouted.

A second doctor looked on quizzically. All of a sudden the anaesthetist seemed less sure of himself. He didn't really know if he should carry on or stop. He didn't find the French doc very inspiring. He stopped for a moment to look at the lines on the monitor. It was showing ventricular fibrillation. Mickey was dying. The anaesthetist started the massage again, with an air of confidence. Arnold couldn't stop himself.

'But he was bradycardic, stable. We have been trying not to lose him for the past hour and now he's in fibrillation because you started heart massage! You don't massage victims of hypothermia.' He added again, 'You're going to kill him.'

Once again the anaesthetist looked a little unsure of what he was doing. In desperation, Arnold turned away so as not to see the rest. He didn't know what else to say, other than, 'Well, you've got to give him cardiac massage now. And there's no point shocking him until you've got his temperature up, it won't work.'

At the same moment, a man was quietly slipping into the resuss room. It was Doctor Polpoth, our Swiss counterpart in the treatment of hypothermia. He is recognized as being one of the top specialists in the field. He is the author of a recent publication cataloguing all the hypothermia cases in cardiac arrest that have been saved by ECC. Thanks to him, we can dare to put the procedure into practice. Yet it will take time to guarantee the efficacy of the system. In a large medical establishment like Geneva hospital, it is far from being accepted as fact. Many practitioners of emergency medicine, excellent though they are, don't have any real understanding of hypothermia cases. There are so many subtleties that the experts still don't understand either.

Continuing his way, and despite Arnold's comments, the young anaesthetist tried placing the paddles of the defibrillator on Mickey's chest and shocking him. His heart started! As if

Doctor Polpoth's entrance had got everything going again. That's what big shots are for!

The animated discussion recommenced. Polpoth, who had come in halfway through, wasn't sure whose side to take. The team was hardly kicking its heels. Arnold had to go, leaving his Swiss colleagues looking a little disconcerted. Polpoth looked puzzled. You shouldn't underestimate the small teams working out in the field with limited resources. The Chamoniards weren't totally devoid of good sense. The size of the hospital wasn't everything.

Three days later Stania was standing at the foot of Mickey's bed. He was still a bit out of it but had certainly perked up a little. He had a cheerful look on his face, even if was still a bit swollen. His fractured pelvis was going to be painful for several months but, for the time being, the worst was his ribs. It was a sneaky kind of pain. Laughing was out of the question!

Stania looked at the small man who had come back from the edge of the abyss and she felt proud to have been part of a miracle. I popped by to say hello. I thought about asking if he had seen a tunnel and a great white light that people who have had near-death experiences talk about. Then I thought better of it. He shouldn't be laughing.

BETTER THAN VEGAS

· · · · · · · · ·

I should have known there'd be something. We were going on holiday the following morning. Sacred, family holidays ... Arco, Italy: pizza, sun, mozzarella, ice cream, the works! It would have been too easy to have spent the evening packing with the kids, checking the tents, sorting out number plates for the trailer and digging out the flippers. That way we could have set off early the next morning, happy to be stress-free.

Instead I had only just got back. The last rescue had left a bitter taste in my mouth. My patient had been in a worse state than it had at first appeared, when I dropped him off at A&E. The call had sounded relatively straightforward: a walker had had a fall on a path and his head was bleeding. He hadn't lost consciousness.

It was Damien at the PGHM who had called me. I was at the hospital looking after a granny who had been taken ill on a walk. Fox had left to fill up.

'Hey, Manu, you coming out to play?' he teased.

'Oh, very funny. What have you got?'

'Walker, head wound. Lot of blood, apparently.'

'Ok, as he's bleeding I might be of some use. Ask Fox if he'd mind very much picking me up from the hospital helipad in five minutes.'

'Ok, I'll call him on the TPH.'

I really like the abbreviations we use, the codes that only we understand. To begin with it seemed like a bit of a laugh, as if we were playing Cowboys and Indians, but I got used to it and it has even crept into the family vocabulary ('Pierrot, stop that or you'll get a WA2LOP!').

We were winched down over the Col des Montets into the scrubby bushes poking up between the rocks. It took a good couple of minutes to find our victim, although he had been easy to spot from above. He was in a patch of wild lettuce, ten metres below the path, sprawled out on a bush, not moving.

His wife didn't seem too distraught. Yet before I had even had time to put my bag down she was assailing me with questions: 'What's the matter with him? Is it serious? Is he bleeding heavily? Is he cold?' I politely asked her to give me two minutes to examine him.

'Are you ok, sir?'

He replied in the affirmative. He was quiet, much quieter than his wife. He instantly had my sympathy. He was trying hard to do as he was told. I was struck by the fact that he seemed to be one of those people who still trusted medics. On the orders of his wife and a passing hiker, he hadn't moved an inch while waiting for the rescue. Every thirty seconds his wife asked him if he was ok and he patiently replied yes.

It sometimes feels like we are arriving at a crime scene. No one wants to touch anything, for fear of destroying possible evidence. He was face down with his nose in a huge lettuce leaf. An impressive gash ran across his head from his forehead to the nape of his neck. And there was a lot of blood! Your scalp is criss-crossed with hundreds of tiny arteries that can bleed a great deal. Especially when no one thinks to staunch the flow. I was surprised no one had tried to stop the bleeding as they waited for us to arrive. His wife, for example. You shouldn't underestimate these kinds of injuries, as you can lose a great deal of blood. Yet given the intravenous therapies at our disposal these days, it would be inconceivable to lose someone this way nowadays …

It was as if his wife had read my mind.

With great tact and sophistication she came out with, 'Is he going to bleed to death?'

It couldn't have been any more indelicate or less conducive to cheering him up if she had asked if I was 'gonna stick him like a pig'.

'He shouldn't do, no. That's why we're here. We'll get him on an IV to replace what he's lost.'

'Lost?'

'The *blood* he's lost.'

'Oh!' And then, shouting a bit too loud for my liking, she said, 'Michel, are you ok?'

She was no doubt convinced that it was imperative in this kind of situation to stop victims from falling asleep in case they died.

'Yes, I'm ok,' he replied, looking more and more out of it.

He just wanted to be left alone.

'Watch out, he wants to be sick!' she suddenly exclaimed, in a worried tone.

She was getting on my nerves. Now it was my turn to be worried.

'Michel, are you ok?'

He was starting to become less responsive. I tried to forget about his wife, who continued to pester me with her questions, and concentrate on the husband. I examined him and he didn't seem to be in pain anywhere else and his neck seemed ok. We sorted ourselves out around him. I placed a large catheter in an obvious-looking vein, ready for the IV. I thought for an instant about giving him a hypertonic solution. But he still had a good peripheral pulse. I opted for a macromolecular solution, as it's better to start off with. I had barely started the injection when he passed out. He had gone very pale and closed his eyes. It was as if I had burst a balloon.

'Michel, are you ok?' his wife asked again.

He was clearly far from ok! However, the IV was flowing. I quickly got out my hypertonic saline solution. We weren't going to lose him like this!

'Michel, are you ok?'

Obviously, in my concern, I too was at an imaginative loss.

'Yes, I'm ok but I think I'm going to be sick,' he said feebly.

That made me feel better. He had already had 300 millilitres and was slowly coming round. His pulse was starting to fluctuate but was still fast. I hadn't even had time to get out my blood pressure cuff. We don't use it that often, as we don't need to know the exact figure in an emergency situation. When a patient's peripheral pulse disappears we know his or her pressure is roughly less than six and we have to get a move on!

Michel was doing better. I didn't know if it was the IV that had saved him or if he had simply had a vasovagal episode, and I preferred to think it had been the latter. We had to get a cervical collar on him. Applying compression bandages to his scalp without moving his neck or taking half the surrounding vegetation with us proved difficult. Despite three successive dressings, blood was still dripping on to the stretcher. We had to do a scoop and run. After a rapid and efficient bit of winching, the helicopter headed straight for Sallanches. On board I tried to staunch the flow of blood from Michel's scalp with my hand. A rivulet of red trickled down along the floor to the front of the helicopter. The EC 145 sped along at 240 kilometres an hour. I saw Chamonix hospital disappear beneath us. Its operating rooms had been closed for bullshit-politico-economic reasons. It seems that small hospitals are dangerous and not economically viable. It was preferable to concentrate the services in Sallanches hospital, twenty-five kilometres down the valley.

And my patient was pissing blood. I hadn't explained to him that he was going to have to bleed for an extra ten minutes so that it would be cheaper for social security. Centralization: the modern malaise! I couldn't help thinking that what we gained on the one hand we lost on the other. We were buying faster and more powerful choppers, but extending the distances they had to fly.

As I dropped off my patient at the A&R I saw that here too they were run off their feet. Every cubicle was occupied, including the resuss room. People were rushing around all over the place. It would have been nice if there had been someone I could talk to, but they obviously had other fish to fry. I was on the verge of taking him up to the operating rooms myself and delivering him into the capable hands of a surgeon. This wasn't the kind of patient you could leave in the corridor. I finally found Fanny, who was standing in as nurse. She took down the details as best she could, rolling her eyes. I just had to hope she would pass them on. She looked exhausted but gave me a friendly smile all the same. That's another flaw with these big institutions: there are always lots of people but never anyone to listen to you!

I got home for dinner, hoping the holidays would start that evening. But at eight-thirty the phone went. I just knew it would.

'Manu, we've got another problem. Can you come to the DZ?'

'Go on, what is it this time?'

'Someone's got their leg stuck in a crack on the Clocheton.'

'Well, just pull it out then!'

'That's what they've been doing, but it won't budge.'

'Ok, I'm on my way.'

I took fifteen seconds to scoff the remains of the stew Cécile had reheated for me, before jumping into the still-warm Subaru. Cécile let out a sigh.

I wasn't happy about having to go in again but it seemed like a slightly daft-sounding rescue mission. And it was warm out and there was a beautiful sunset.

There was a great deal of activity at the DZ. They had got out the ironmongery: oil can, generator, drill. Somebody handed me a plastic bag full of ice cubes, which I stared at blankly.

'He's been there for a few hours, we thought it might reduce the swelling in his leg …'

I wasn't convinced but took the bag all the same. No point complaining. Laurent and Tintin were already there. Zeb and Filou were getting ready to take the generator up and give a hand. They had thought of everything, even floodlights, as it was getting dark. It was going to be like Las Vegas up there! While Fox's engine started up I tried to imagine the scene: the bloke with his leg caught in the crack, like a rat in a trap, on top of the Clocheton.

The Clocheton du Brévent is a short but classic old-style route. It's great for people who want to do a minimum of climbing and a maximum of ropework: abseils into space, throwing the rope, a Tyrolean traverse … The Clocheton itself is a small, fifty-metre spike of rock poking up out of the Aiguilles Rouges. The top tapers to a point and there isn't even enough room for a bivouac. You can throw a rope over a spike and cross on to its sister peak a few dozen metres away.

Fox took off. I sat in the back, digesting my stew. What could I do for the poor bloke? I'm a doctor not a quarryman! I certainly wasn't going to embark on some kind of impromptu cowboy amputation. I hoped it would sort itself out without too much damage.

I have learned to be prepared. We set off without a care in the world, expecting a walk in the park, and we end up slogging our guts out for whole nights at a time, like coal miners. I had taken a warm jacket and some Ketamine, my weapon of choice. The Clocheton finally poked its nose up into the pale shades of the horizon as night was falling. I got ready to be lowered down.

First, attach my bag to the loop on my harness. I was miles away that night, as I did everything the wrong way round. The usual routine had changed with the arrival of the new helicopter. It was very straightforward in training but the slightest mistake on a mission and you were liable to cock everything up. I clipped the safety sling into the steel ring that goes round the loop on my harness and moved towards Chris, the mechanic. He gestured to me. It was time to go down. Fox was perfectly stationary, not budging an inch. I sat on the edge. Chris held out the winch for me and I clipped it to the steel ring. The machine effortlessly winched me out and I turned round, my arse in space.

Cock-up number one: despite being in the job for fifteen years, I had forgotten to take off my headset. A classic mistake! The cable tugged at me. Chris gave me a look. He couldn't bear people wrecking his gear. Cock-up number two: my bag was caught underneath the first sling and I had a hell of a job to free it. Then I realized I hadn't brought the right gloves with me and I couldn't feel what I was doing. Things were going pear-shaped. But whatever we did we couldn't undo the winch, as there might be unpleasant consequences. Chris kept the cable tight. It took a bit of work but I finally managed to disentangle myself.

I was moving away from the cabin on the arm of the winch. I was dangling beneath the rotor blades, above the Clocheton. I finally dared look at the spectacle below. I was right: it did look like Vegas! The red and green lights of the chopper and the floodlights at the bottom of the tapering pinnacle with four figures suspended from it, made the scene look even more bizarre than I had expected.

The Clocheton's prisoner, an Australian, was well and truly wedged up to his thigh in the final crack. Around fifteen metres higher up Zeb sat astride the summit. Tintin was hanging beneath him, next to the stranded climber. I arrived right above them. As I whirled round, I caught Tintin's hand and he pulled me towards the only bolt, to which he had already clipped himself. Below us lay nothing but air. Thankfully, Zeb had everybody on a back up, with two ropes he had attached to his stance. The big bumble-bee winched the gear down to us and flew off. After the tornado came silence. I suddenly realized how much I liked doing rescues this way. It was a sufficiently rare occurrence for me to say so.

'This is great, we should do this more often!' I shouted.

There was no response from the others. They were already deep in concentration.

The Australian definitely wasn't enjoying himself but didn't seem to understand French. The expression on his face was a mixture of concern and hope. I explained that I was a doctor. Not only did he look like he didn't believe me, but I could also tell that he had no idea how I was going to get him out of there. No doubt he would have preferred a high-explosive specialist!

We started by giving him a warm duvet jacket, as he had been trapped in his shorts for over three hours and was freezing his arse off. I pictured what had happened. His girlfriend, belaying him thirty metres below, couldn't have seen him get his leg stuck. He had wedged himself further in as he tried to pull himself free. It had taken her a while to realize what had happened. She managed to abseil down, thanks to the second rope they had thought to bring. She then ran to the Brévent lift to get help.

Tintin outlined the situation to me. The Australian's leg was bent and his thigh trapped in a crack no more than thirty centimetres wide. They had tried pulling him from above, but it hadn't worked. I brought the oil. We poured the whole can over his thigh. His shorts were covered in it, but he didn't mind. The next climber on the route would have been wise to avoid the crack and its slippery holds.

We had another go. We tried hauling him, attaching jumars right, left and centre. He didn't budge. The guy wriggled and pulled at his leg, but the more we pulled, the more jammed he became. John – for that was his name – remained stuck fast. I was already considering our more aggressive plans of action. The first consisted in giving him a shot of something so that we could pull him out with the cable winch. It might make him scream a bit! I opened my bag. I'm quite proud of the fact that its wallet-style design makes it ideal for this kind of situation: nothing falls out and I have everything I need on my left-hand side while I can treat my patient to my right. Suspended in mid-air, I placed the traditional catheter and cap in his forearm, while Tintin prepared the syringe for me. As I injected him, I explained that the drug was like morphine and it would help him to relax. I didn't dare tell him we were going to heave him out like an old nag!

We now had to wait for the rest of the gear that we could hear coming up from the valley floor. The bumble-bee was back, no more musical than before. Again it hovered, stationary, above our heads, the rotor blades skimming over the Clocheton in the night. The floodlights illuminated the gneiss. It made a beautiful spectacle. I was surprised by how precise the winching at night had been. Everything was brought up to a plateau. The bumble-bee flew off. We started work again.

Filou sorted out the generator that had been dropped off lower down, at a small col, while Zeb and Laurent set up the Paillardet winch on the top of the Clocheton. I wondered how they were going to manage on such a small platform. At the same time, the drill was being lowered down to us. We might be able to dislodge the flake of rock that was trapping his leg at the level of his knee. I passed the extension lead down to Filou, fifteen metres below. It was just long enough, without a metre to spare. The generator started up. It was disappointing to begin with. The drill wriggled around like a sardine but had no power, barely enough to dislodge the lichen. I saw how thick the granite was. What's more, whenever we applied any pressure, the generator choked up. I was starting to wonder how effective we would actually be. Other, more radical, solutions were taking shape in my mind: a Kétalar injection and a sharp tug with the Paillardet and its steel cable? What would that achieve? We'd wreck his knee. Why not take off the whole leg while we were at it. I could already see the headlines in the local paper. 'First there was *Jaws*, now the mountains have teeth: ravenous crack tears leg off unconscious climber!' We couldn't let that happen, it really wouldn't be very professional …

'Oi, Filou, can't you turn up the gas? We've got bugger all coming out up here.'

'It's on maximum,' replied Filou.

Tintin persevered, trying from every possible angle. I watched him, not convinced, waiting for him to say, 'Stupid-bloody-shitty-drill!'

But suddenly it gave way. The sliver of granite trapping the climber's knee split open. Tintin held it between two fingers and pulled. And that was it. As if by some miracle, the whole flake came away in his hand. Tintin slid the lump of rock out and gave me a look, a glint in his eye. John moved his leg and bent it back and forth with disconcerting ease. The sense of relief was palpable. He was swimming in a mixture of morphine- and release-induced elation. Tintin was shouting at the top of his lungs, as if he had scored the winning goal in a cup final. He was more pleased than the Australian!

'Did you see that, lads? You can put your tools away, doc. You won't need them tonight. It's only midnight, you're gonna be able to go on holiday after all!'

EPILOGUE

• • • • • • • • •

The road seemed to go on for ever, up the endless twists and turns to Plateau d'Assy. It was autumn, it was raining. I had come back from an expedition to Nepal completely jetlagged but relaxed. I need these breaks in the back of beyond to recover, to shake off the burden, which hours of being on call builds up inside me.

Ratna Chuli, which we had climbed, is a beautiful peak. If one is to believe the significantly different heights given on the various maps of the area, it must be somewhere around the 7,000-metre mark. Unlike the previous peak we had attempted, this time we were successful. Thanks to exceptional weather conditions and extraordinary views across the Tibetan plateau, we had come away with lasting memories.

As usual, I had had to face the eternal problems of expedition medicine, mostly to do with acclimatization. There had been nothing really serious that year, just a pulmonary oedema at base camp. We set about treating it with gusto, thanks to the HAPE-specific drugs I had taken care to add to my kit and, more importantly, thanks to the portable recompression bag we always carry with us on trips.

I made the most of a free day when we got back to Kathmandu to go and see Khando. I had been careful not to let her know I was coming just in case I couldn't make it and to keep it as a surprise. Khando was at school, Mount Kailash High School, perched on top of a small hill. She came up to me, shy but happy. She was squeezed into her school uniform: small green V-neck jumper, grey pleated skirt, short white blouse and tiny skew-whiff black tie. The outfit was second-hand but smelt heavily of washing powder. We hugged each other tightly. After that, not really knowing what to say, Khando took me on a tour of the school, which was very nice.

I was relieved. Khando had a bit of a cry when I left but I knew she was doing fine. I insisted she work particularly hard on her English. I explained that if we could be patient for a little while longer she would be able to come to the Ecole de Taconnaz on a more regular basis. Thanks to the Tibetan school, I now knew that Khando's stays in France would be easier to organize.

I parked in the huge car park at the rehab centre in Plateau d'Assy. I was early. The scene that greeted me in the entrance hall immediately set the tone. Two guys in wheelchairs were chatting by the lift and a tired-looking young woman smoking a cigarette was daydreaming by the window. She was holding an IV-line on a lead and it looked like her sole companion. A grandmother shuffled uncomfortably down the corridor, leaning on a young man with a beard and a white coat.

I asked for the room number I needed at reception and went up to the second floor. As I neared the door I slowed down. I hesitated for a moment: what was I going to say? I had so little and yet so much to say. Curiously, I was a little afraid and, taking a deep breath, I knocked on the door.

Jarvis, the skier who had jumped thirty metres over a cliff and whose broken body we had struggled to hold together in the end of last winter's dusk, was near the window, quietly sitting in an armchair, a book on his knees. I would never have recognized him. I wondered for an instant if I had got the wrong room. The guy had been dead: it was inconceivable to think that this face could have an expression, an identity.

He gave me a calm yet questioning look. I was going to have to tell him his own story ... Our story!